Allergy and Asthma

made ridiculously simple

Massoud Mahmoudi, DO, PhD, FACOI, FAOCAI, FACP, FCCP, FAAAAI

President
American Osteopathic College of
Allergy and Immunology

Associate Clinical Professor
Department of Medicine
University of California–San Francisco
San Francisco, California

Clinical Professor
Department of Medicine
School of Osteopathic Medicine
Rowan University
Stratford, New Jersey

Adjunct Associate Professor
Department of Medicine
San Francisco College of Osteopathic Medicine
Touro University
Vallejo, California

Editor/Author of:
Challenging Cases in Allergy and Immunology, Humana Press, 2009
Challenging Cases in Allergic and Immunologic Disease of the Skin, Springer, 2010
Challenging Cases in Pulmonology, Springer, 2011
Challenging Cases in Rheumatology and Diseases of the Immune System, Springer, 2012
Allergy and Asthma: Practical Diagnosis and Management (Ed-2), Springer, 2016

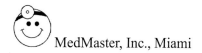 MedMaster, Inc., Miami

ISBN 10 #1-935660-25-X
ISBN 13 #978-1-935660-25-5

Made in the United States of America

Published by
MedMaster, Inc.
P.O. Box 640028
Miami, FL 33164
www.mmbks@aol.com

Cover image by Richard March

*To the memory of my father, Mohammad H. Mahmoudi,
and to my mother, Zohreh, my wife, Lily, and
my sons, Sam and Sina, for their sincere
support and encouragement.*

Preface

It is a pleasure to introduce "Allergy and Asthma Made Ridiculously Simple" to the family of the "MedMaster" book series. This book follows the same format as my predecessor book "Immunology Made Ridiculously Simple."

As in the other publications by MedMaster, this book emphasizes the more relevant clinical information for the students of medicine. The more detailed information in some parts of the book is for clarification and better understanding of the subject.

This book covers all aspects of allergic disease and asthma in a simplified format. Allergies affect most organ systems of the body; some patients suffer from allergic rhinitis, some from asthma, and others from skin allergies such as eczema (atopic dermatitis), urticaria/angioedema, and allergic contact dermatitis. Basic inquiry about allergies (such as drug or latex) should be part of every patient history regardless of chief complaint. More detailed questions are reserved for the allergic patient.

The importance of understanding allergic diseases and asthma is clear, when more than 50 million people suffer from allergies in the United States each year. In addition to the suffering, the cost of management is estimated to be over 18 billion dollars per year due to the use of medications, emergency treatment, and loss of school or workdays.

This book consists of 11 chapters starting with an introduction to the immune system and ending with immunotherapy, followed by an Appendix with the common questions useful for taking a history from an allergic patient.

This is an introductory course intended for medical students, residents, primary care providers, nursing students, nurses, nurse practitioners and allied health majors as well as other clinicians who want to learn the practical aspects of evaluating and treating allergic patients. This is not a Board prep. To complement the presented book, I encourage you to review " Immunology Made Ridiculously Simple" for more details of the immune system.

This book of the series, like the other members of the MedMaster family, benefited from the guidance of Dr. Stephen Goldberg, the author, educator and the publisher of the series. He has guided me by close involvement in preparation of the book to ensure the standard of the series for the last 37 years.

I am indebted to Dr. Goldberg for this opportunity to use this medium to share what I know about the subject. I also would like to express my gratitude to Phyllis Goldenberg for the proofreading and to Richard March for the cover design. I also thank Professor Satoshi Yoshida for sharing some the derm-related photos of his collection that I have used for a better clarification of the subjects.

As always I welcome your comments and feedback to use for the future editions. Please feel free contact me at allergycure@sbcglobal.net.

Contents

Chapter 1
The World of Allergy

An allergen is a substance that triggers a pathological hypersensitive immune response called an *allergic reaction.*

The five main categories of allergens are *environmental* (indoor/outdoor), *food, drug, occupational,* and *cosmetic.* However, many allergens do not belong to any specific categories (**Fig. 1-1**).

FIGURE 1-1. TYPES OF ALLERGENS	
ALLERGEN TYPES	**EXAMPLES**
Environmental (Outdoor)	• Trees (juniper, cedar, cyprus) • Grasses (Johnson, Timothy, meadow fescue) • Weeds (ragweed; lamb's quarter) • Insects (yellow jacket; honey bee)
Environmental (Indoor)	• Dust mites (Dermatophagoides farinae; Dermatophagoides pteronyssinus) • Pets (cats, dogs) • Molds (Penicillium, Alternaria, Cladosporium) • Cockroaches
Food	• Peanuts • Tree nuts • Shellfish (shrimp)
Drug	Penicillin; neomycin
Occupational	Latex
Cosmetic	• Perfumes • Nail polish
Others	Glue

ENVIRONMENTAL ALLERGENS

There are two types of environmental allergens: *outdoor allergens* and *indoor allergens.* Outdoor allergens include pollens (trees, grasses, and weeds) and insects (Vespids: bee family). Indoor allergens include dust mites, pets, molds, and cockroaches.

Outdoor Allergens

Trees. Tree pollens are one of the common outdoor allergens. Trees become problematic during the pollinating season. Usually, tree pollens are loose; a mild wind can remove them from the trees. These airborne allergens are easily inhaled by affected individuals who happen to be outdoors. Interestingly, the trees with pretty flowers are not a direct source of an allergic reaction because their pollens are transported by insects. As a result, they are rarely aerosolized and available in the air. Although the pollinating seasons differ from one region to another, trees (as a rule of thumb) pollinate in the spring.

Grasses. Usually there is a structural homology among grasses, and individuals who are allergic to one specific grass (e.g. Timothy) commonly react to other grasses (e.g. meadow fescue). Some grasses, such as Johnson grass, have a unique structure and do not cross react with other grasses. Again, depending on region, pollinating seasons may differ, but grasses usually pollinate in the summer.

Weeds. Some weeds share a structural homology as well. Although weeds differ in various regions, some, such as ragweeds, are abundant in many parts of the United States. Weeds pollinate in later summer and early fall.

Stinging Insects. To simplify, there are three families of stinging insects: **Apidae** (honey bee, bumblebee, and sweetbee), **Vespidae** (yellow jacket, yellow hornet, white-faced hornet and paper wasp) and **Formicidae** (fire ants and harvester ant) (**Fig. 1-2**).

FIGURE 1-2. STINGING INSECTS	
STINGING INSECTS (FAMILY)	**NAME**
Apidae	Honeybee Bumblebee Sweetbee
Vespidae	Yellow jacket Yellow hornet White-faced hornet Paper wasp
Formicidae	Fire ant Harvester ant

Indoor Allergens

Dust Mites. These 8-legged sightless microscopic organisms feed on organic matter such as scales of human skin or feathers. Two of the common dust mites are *Dermatophagoides* *farina* (*D. f*) and *Dermatophagoides pteronyssinus* (*D. pt*). They enjoy living in a humid environment (over 50% humidity), which is actually a must for their survival.

Pets. Many animals live inside as pets. The most common source of pet allergens is cats. The major cat allergen is Fel d1.

Molds. Molds originate outdoors, but they can find their way indoors and settle in damp and humid areas of the house. Prolonged inhalation of mold spores can make the susceptible individual sensitized and allergic. Examples of indoor molds are *Penicillium, Alternaria,* and *Cladosporium.*

Cockroaches. Several species of cockroaches live in a household environment. Two are *Blattella germanica* (German cockroach) and *Periplaneta americana* (American cockroach). What makes their indoor allergens important is their relationship with asthma. In a study of asthmatics who presented to inner city emergency rooms, the source of their asthma triggers was traced to cockroach-infested residences.

ALLERGIES BY ORGAN SYSTEM

For an allergic reaction to occur, an allergen should eventually find its way to the mast cells, which are located in connective tissue throughout the body. The ports of entry of allergens are the skin, mucous membranes, and upper airways (mouth and nares) (**Fig. 1-3**).

FIGURE 1-3. PORTS OF ALLERGEN ENTRANCE		
PORT OF ENTRY	**EXAMPLES OF AFFECTED AREAS**	**EXAMPLES OF AN ALLERGIC REACTION**
Skin	Palms	Allergic contact dermatitis; urticaria
Mucous membranes	Conjunctiva	Allergic conjunctivitis
Oropharynx	Lips, tongue	Angioedema
Oropharynx	Larynx	Laryngeoedema
Nares	Turbinates	Allergic rhinitis

One type of allergen may enter the host by different routes. For example, food can enter the body via the oropharynx or by exposure to the skin. Drugs can enter the host by ingestion, skin absorption, or direct inoculation (injections: subcutaneous, intradermal, intramuscular, or intravenous) (**Fig. 1-4**).

One common way of classifying allergic diseases is by the affected target organ/system (**Fig. 1-5**):

FIGURE 1-4. ENTRANCE OF PARTICULAR ALLERGENS INTO THE HOST					
TYPE OF ALLERGEN	**SKIN**	**MUCOUS MEMBRANE**	**ORAL**	**NARES**	**BLOOD**
Pollen		+		+	
Insect	+				
Food	+	+	+		
Drug	+	+	+	+	+
Cosmetics	+	+			

FIGURE 1-5. CLASSIFICATION OF ALLERGIC DISEASES BASED ON TARGET ORGAN	
AFFECTED ANATOMY	**EXAMPLES OF ALLERGIC DISEASE**
Eyes	Allergic conjunctivitis
Ears	Eczema; allergic contact dermatitis
Nose	Allergic rhinitis
Eyes and nose	Allergic rhinoconjunctivitis
Lungs	Asthma
Skin	Atopic dermatitis
Skin	Urticaria; angioedema
Skin	Allergic contact dermatitis

Allergic Diseases of the Eyes

An allergic reaction may occur in areas around the eye (*periorbital*); such reactions include *angioedema* (angio: blood vessel; edema: inflammation) or allergic contact dermatitis.

The conjunctiva (**Fig. 1-6**), which lines the inner eyelid and the front surface of the eye up to the cornea, may also be the target of an allergen invasion (*allergic conjunctivitis*).

Allergic Diseases of the Ears

Eczema. The external ear structure may become eczematous; these areas of skin are inflamed, excoriated, and pruritic.

Allergic contact dermatitis. Certain hearing aids may cause allergic contact dermatitis.

Allergic Diseases of the Nose

The most common allergy of the nose is *allergic rhinitis* (rhino: nose + itis: inflammation). Although allergic rhinitis literally means allergic nose (inflamed nose), by definition, allergic rhinitis is a constellation of various symptoms, including nasal congestion, rhinorrhea, sneezing, itchy palate, etc., which are collectively referred to as allergic rhinitis. (See more details in later chapters.)

THE CONJUNCTIVA

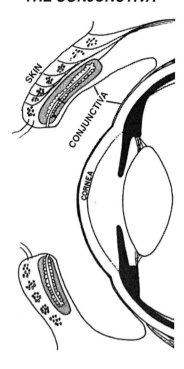

FIGURE 1-6. (From Goldberg, S. and Trattler, W. Ophthalmology Made Ridiculously Simple, Medmaster)

Allergic Asthma

Asthma is a chronic reversible inflammatory disease of the airways. The most common type of asthma is *allergic asthma*, which results after repeated exposure to aeroallergens.

Systemic Reaction (Anaphylaxis)

Anaphylaxis is an acute and life-threatening allergic reaction to an allergen, which causes multi-organ failure. Anaphylaxis may be fatal if not recognized and treated immediately.

Allergic Diseases of the Skin

- *Atopic dermatitis* is a condition in which affected individuals have eczema and are atopic (genetically have a predisposition to allergies).
- *Urticaria* is an allergic skin condition in which the affected area becomes inflamed and pruritic.
- *Angioedema* is an allergic skin condition in which the affected area becomes inflamed and swollen, with a burning sensation. The affected areas are usually mucous membranes, periorbital areas, lips, tongue, larynx (*laryngioedema*), lining of the gut, hands and genitalia.
- *Allergic contact dermatitis* is a delayed allergic reaction that results from contact with an allergen such as poison oak, cosmetics, jewelry, and some drugs.

Chapter 2
Four Classes of Hypersensitivity

Allergic reactions can generally be broken up into four types, according to the Gell-Coombs classification: *Types I, II, III,* and *IV* (**Fig. 2-1**):

FIGURE 2-1. GELL AND COOMBS CLASSIFICATION OF HYPERSENSITIVITY REACTIONS	
TYPE OF HYPERSENSI-TIVITY REACTION	**ALSO KNOWN AS**
Type I	Immediate hypersensitivity, anaphylactic, or IgE-mediated
Type II	Antibody (IgG or IgM) mediated
Type III	Immune complex-mediated
Type IV	Cell-mediated or delayed type

TYPE I HYPERSENSITIVITY (IgE-MEDIATED)

Immunoglobulins (also called *antibodies*) are glycoproteins produced by plasma cells in response to antigens, which are foreign microbial and non-microbial substances. There are 5 different isotypes (classes) of immunoglobulins: *IgG, IgA, IgM, IgE,* and *IgD*. The mnemonic GAMED helps to remember them (**Fig. 2-2**).

IgE has the shortest half-life (2.5 days) among the immunoglobulins. IgE is produced in response to a specific allergen. IgE binds to high affinity receptors on *mast cells* and *basophils*, inducing *degranulation,* the release of mast cell and basophil *mediators* of the allergic reaction (**Figs. 2-3, 2-4, 2-5**), with attending local vasodilatation, vascular

FEATURES OF IMMUNOGLOBULINS

Immunoglobulin	Structure	Function
IgG	monomer	prominent in secondary response
IgA	dimer (J-chain)	prominent in secretions
IgM	pentamer	prominent in primary antibody response
IgE	long Fc fragment	prominent in worm infestations & allergies. Binds to Fc receptors on mast cells and basophils, causing them to release inflammatory substances
IgD	monomer	receptor on B-lymphocytes

FIGURE 2-2. (From Mahmoudi, M. Immunology Made Ridiculously Simple, Medmaster)

permeability, edema, inflammation and, at times, systemic reactions, with multi-organ involvement (*anaphylaxis*).

FIGURE 2-3. FEATURES OF MAST CELLS (From Mahmoudi, M. Immunology Made Ridiculously Simple, Medmaster)	
Feature	Characteristic
Origin	Bone marrow
Size	10-15 µm
Nucleus	Bilobed or multilobed
Distribution	Skin and connective tissues
Morphologic distinction under light microscope	Purplish color due to stained granules
Half-life	Weeks to months
Examples of cytoplasmic granule contents	Histamine, heparin chondroitin sulfate, proteases
Function	• One of the main effector cells in immediate hypersensitivity • Produces wheal and flare by releasing histamine

FIGURE 2-4. FEATURES OF BASOPHILS (From Mahmoudi, M. Immunology Made Ridiculously Simple, Medmaster)	
Feature	Characteristic
Origin	Bone marrow
Cell type	Granulocyte
Size	12-15 µm
Nucleus	Multilobed
Distribution	Peripheral blood, tissues
Morphologic distinction under light microscope	Multilobed nucleus, bluish color when stained with the basic dye, methylene blue
Half-life	Days
Cytoplasmic granule contents	Histamine, Major Basic Protein, Charcot-Leyden protein, chondroitin sulfate, neutral proteinases. leukotriene C4, TNF-alpha, IL-4
Function	• It is one of the effector cells in immediate hypersensitivity. • It also participates in the late phase reaction of allergic response.

Common Mediators in Mast Cells and Basophils

Secretory protein	Type of protein	Functions
Histamine	Vasoactive amines	• Vasodilates, increases vascular permeability • Bronchospasm
Neutral proteases (Tryptase, chymase carboxypeptidase, cathepsin)	Enzyme	• Degrades tissues • Damages microbial structures
Chondroitin Sulfate	Proteoglycan	Participates in structural matrix of granules
Platelet-activating factor	Lipid mediator	• Attracts leukocytes • Increases vascular permeability • Activates neutrophils, eosinophils, and platelets • Bronchoconstricts
Leukotriene C4 (LTC4), D4 (LTD4), and E4 (LTE4)	Lipid mediator	• Bronchospasm • Increases vascular permeability and constriction of arterial, arteriolar, and intestinal smooth muscle
Prostaglandin D2 (PGD2)	Lipid mediator	• Vasodilates • Increases vascular permeability • Bronchoconstricts • Inhibits platelet aggregation • Stimulates neutrophil chemotaxis (attracts neutrophils)
TNF-α	Cytokines	Activates neutrophils
IL-4	Cytokines	• Promotes TH2 differentiation, isotype switching to IgE • B cell proliferation • Eosinophil and mast cell growth and function
IL-5	Cytokines	• Stimulates eosinophil production, activation, growth, and differentiation • Stimulates B lymphocyte proliferation
IL-6	Cytokines	Induces fever, acute phase response (liver)
IL-13	Cytokines	Similar to IL-4

FIGURE 2-5. (From Mahmoudi, M. Immunology Made Ridiculously Simple, Medmaster)

Mast cells and basophils originate in the bone marrow. Undifferentiated mast cells enter the blood circulation and differentiate upon arriving at the tissues. They reside in the skin, connective tissue, and mucosal epithelium of the gastrointestinal, urinary, and respiratory tracts. Basophils reside in the peripheral blood.

Both mast cells and basophils have high affinity receptors (*FcεRI*) on their cell surfaces, which are targets of IgE antibody binding, and both cells types release histamine and other inflammatory mediators.

Type I hypersensitivity reactions proceed according to the following steps (**Fig. 2-6**):

A. Exposure of the host (B lymphocyte cells, antigen-presenting cells) to an allergen (such as tree pollen or dust mites).

B. The activated B cells bind to Th2 (T-helper) cells (a type of lymphocyte), which become activated.

C. B cells undergo *class switching* (production of a different class of antibodies than the B cell would otherwise produce, with different functions) and produce a specific IgE to the allergen.

D. IgE binds to the high affinity *FcεRI* receptors on the mast or basophil cell surface.

E. Re-exposure to the allergen.

F. Mast cell and basophil degranulation occur, with release of various inflammatory mediators, including histamine.

G. Vasodilation, vascular permeability, edema, and inflammation.

Examples of Type I hypersensitivity range from the annoyance of pollen allergy to anaphylaxis from certain foods. The allergist is most concerned with Type I hypersensitivity.

TYPE II HYPERSENSITIVITY (IgG- or IgM-MEDIATED)

Type II Hypersensitivity, like Type I hypersensitivity, is antibody-mediated but is the result of an interaction between IgG or IgM with an antigen (cell surface or an extracellular matrix antigen).

There are three ways in which the antigens are destroyed:

MECHANISM OF TYPE I HYPERSENSITIVITY REACTIONS

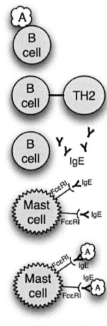

- Exposure of the host (B cells, antigen presenting cell) to the allergen (A)

- Binding of the activated B cells to TH2 (T-helper) cells and activation of the TH2 cells

- B cells undergo class switching to antibody-producing (IgE) cells; production of specific IgE to the allergen A

- Binding of the IgE to high affinity receptor FcεRI on mast cells

- Re-exposure to the allergen A

- Mast cell degranulation and release of various mediators, including histamine, prostaglandins, leukotrienes, and others

- Vasodilation, vascular permeability, edema

Histamine

FIGURE 2-6. (From Mahmoudi, M. Immunology Made Ridiculously Simple, Medmaster)

1. *Opsonization* and *phagocytosis*. In *opsonization*, the binding of an antibody to an antigen becomes a target for phagocytosis (**Fig. 2-7**).

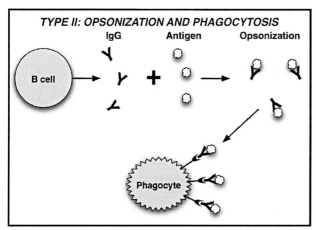

FIGURE 2-7. (From Mahmoudi, M. Immunology Made Ridiculously Simple, Medmaster)

2. *Antibody-dependent cellular toxicity (ADCC)*. First, an IgG binds to surface of an infected cell; then the IgG-infected cell complex is recognized and destroyed by NK (Natural Killer) cells (**Fig. 2-8**).

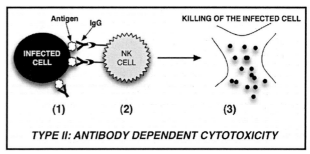

FIGURE 2-8. (From Mahmoudi, M. Immunology Made Ridiculously Simple, Medmaster)

3. *Complement activation*. Complement is a group of plasma proteins that is integral to the immune response.

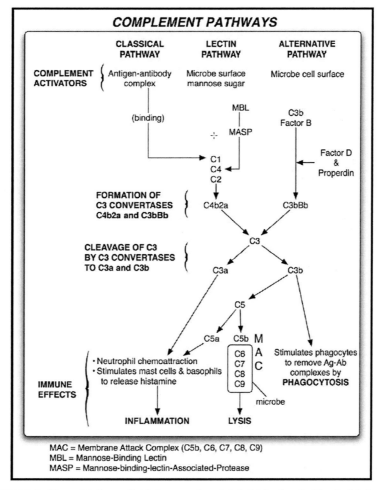

FIGURE 2-9. (From Mahmoudi, M. Immunology Made Ridiculously Simple, Medmaster)

When complement is activated by an antigen-antibody complex, there are a cascading series of reactions ending in phagocytosis and lysis of bacteria. Activated complement also stimulates mast cells and basophils to release histamine (**Fig. 2-9**), as well as neutrophil chemoattraction, thus promoting inflammation.

Destruction of allergens in Type II hypersensitivity reaction can harm the host for two reasons. First, microbial antigens sometimes persist, and their destruction causes inflammation and injury. Second, the body sometimes fails to distinguish self from nonself, and the antibody attacks the body, causing an autoimmune disease.

Examples of Type II drug sensitivity include hemolytic anemia (e.g. from penicillin), thrombocytopenia, and neutropenia.

TYPE III HYPERSENSITIVITY (IMMUNE COMPLEX-MEDIATED)

In *Type III hypersensitivity*, binding of an antigen and an antibody forms an immune complex. This complex either activates the complement system and is phagocytized or it escapes and the immune complex precipitates in various anatomical sites, causing, for example, vasculitis in blood vessels, nephritis in the kidney, and arthritis in the synovial joints. The prototype of Type III hypersensitivity reactions is sickness that may develop 4-21 days (usually 8-10) days after administration of a drug such as penicillin. Other examples are drug fever and vasculitis (**Fig. 2-10**).

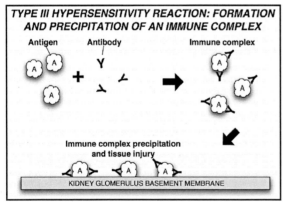

TYPE III HYPERSENSITIVITY REACTION: FORMATION AND PRECIPITATION OF AN IMMUNE COMPLEX

Antigen   Antibody   Immune complex

Immune complex precipitation and tissue injury

KIDNEY GLOMERULUS BASEMENT MEMBRANE

FIGURE 2-10. (From Mahmoudi, M. Immunology Made Ridiculously Simple, Medmaster)

TYPE IV HYPERSENSITIVITY (CELL-MEDIATED; DELAYED)

The major players of Type IV hypersensitivity are T cells. T cells are lymphocytes and are part of adaptive immunity (a system of host defense that possesses memory and can distinguish specific antigens). The two major subtypes of T cells are CD4+ helper T cells and CD8+ cytotoxic T cells.

Type IV hypersensitivity results from an interaction between antigens (presented by antigen-presenting cells) and T lymphocyte cells (CD4+ helper T cells and CD8+ cytotoxic T cells). Binding of antigens to T cells activates the T cells, which then release cytokines such as IFN-gamma, leading to tissue inflammation and injury (**Fig. 2-11**). CD8+ cytotoxic T lymphocytes can also directly kill the infected target cells (**Fig. 2-11**).

TYPE IV HYPERSENSITIVITY

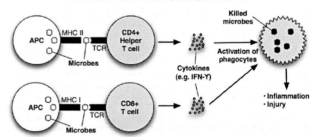

CD4+ HELPER T CELLS, CD8+ T CELLS AND CELL-MEDIATED HYPERSENSITIVITY REACTIONS

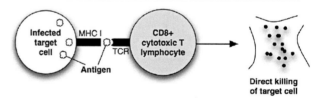

DIRECT KILLING OF INFECTED TARGET CELLS BY CD8+ CYTOTOXIC T LYMPHOCYTES

FIGURE 2-11. (From Mahmoudi, M. Immunology Made Ridiculously Simple, Medmaster)

Chapter 3
Allergic Diseases of the Eye

ALLERGIC CONJUNCTIVITIS

The patient with allergic conjunctivitis commonly presents with complaints of red, itchy, and watery eyes. Sometimes, conjunctivitis is associated with nasal symptoms (rhinitis), a problem collectively termed *allergic rhinoconjunctivitis.* Other symptoms of allergic conjunctivitis include burning, stinging, and photophobia; however, itching is the most common symptom (**Fig. 3-1**). The affected individual may become symptomatic during a transient exposure to an allergen (*acute allergic conjunctivitis*), during a specific season (*seasonal allergic conjunctivitis*) or all year (*perennial allergic conjunctivitis*). The difference between the last two groups is the type of allergen involved and the duration of the symptoms. In seasonal allergic conjunctivitis, the involved allergens are pollens but in perennial allergic conjunctivitis, the allergens are those that are available throughout the year, such as dust mites or pet dander (**Fig. 1-1**).

FIGURE 3-1. CHARACTERISTICS OF ALLERGIC CONJUNCTIVITIS	
Symptoms	Red, watery, itching, burning eyes, photophobia
Types	Seasonal or perennial
Sex Preference	None
Visual Damage	None
Prevalence	Common
Other associated symptoms	Occasionally associated with shiner (black eye)

The allergic symptoms are the result of direct contact between the conjunctiva and the aeroallergens. Repeated exposure of the allergen to the conjunctiva stimulates the sensitized mast cells, causing degranulation and release of histamine and other chemical mediators. The mechanism of the allergic reaction is basically similar to that of allergic rhinitis.

Diagnosis of Allergic Conjunctivitis

Inspection of the eyes should include the conjunctiva, eyelids, and periorbital areas. Are both eyes involved (more likely in allergy)? Is the conjunctiva dry (as in Sjogren's syndrome – see below)? Is there any discharge? If so, is the discharge watery and clear (suggestive of viral or allergic etiology)? Is there any swelling of the eyelids? Is there a *shiner* (a "black eye" shadow underneath the eyes, suggesting allergy)?

If the presenting eye symptoms are associated with nasal symptoms, then the examiner should consider an allergy *prick test (*an allergy skin test in which allergens are pricked into the skin with a needle-like device to stimulate an allergic response) to investigate the presence of IgE antibody to indoor or outdoor allergens.

Treatment of Allergic Conjunctivitis

The extent of treatment depends on the level, duration, and frequency of allergen exposure and finally the intensity of the reaction.

Non-pharmacological Treatment of Allergic Conjunctivitis:

The best strategy to avoid the allergic symptoms is to avoid exposure to allergens. For example, on a windy day with high pollen count, the best remedy is to stay indoors.

Pharmacological Treatment of Allergic Conjunctivitis:

- *Antihistamines.* Topical eye drops (e.g. *emedastine*) are preferred over oral medication for allergic conjunctivitis. However, if nasal symptoms are present, consider oral antihistamines or both oral and ophthalmic routes if needed (**Fig. 3-2**).

- *Mast Cell Stabilizers.* Use of topical eye drops (e.g. *cromolyn*) is preferred over oral medication for allergic conjunctivitis. However, if nasal symptoms are present, consider an oral antihistamine or both if needed.

- *Antihistamine/Mast Cell Stabilizers.* These topical medications (e.g. *olopatadine*) have two mechanisms of action and therefore are more potent than a single action drug.

- *Vasoconstrictors.* Prolonged use of this class of medication is not recommended, because the medication loses its efficacy and may cause a rebound of symptoms upon cessation (*conjunctivitis medicamentosa*).

CLASS	GENERIC (BRAND NAME) EXAMPLES	DOSAGE
Antihistamines	emedastine (Emadine)	≥ 3 years: 1 drop up to 4 times a day
Mast cell stabilizer	pemirolast (Alamast)	≥ 3 years: 1-2 drops 4 times a day
	cromolyn sodium (Crolom)	≥ 4 years: 1-2 drops 4-6 times a day
	nedocromil (Alocril)	≥ 3 years: 1-2 drops 2 times a day
Antihistamine-mast cell stabilizer	azelastine (Optivar)	≥ 3 years: 1 drop twice a day
	olopatadine (Patanol)	≥ 3 years: 1 drop twice a day (6-8 hours apart)
	ketotifen (Zaditor)	≥ 3 years: 1 drop every 8-12 hours, max: 2 doses a day
Vasoconstrictors	naphazoline	1 or 2 drops every 3-4 hours a day
Antihistamine +vasoconstrictor	naphazoline+ pheniramine (Naphcon A)	≥ 6 years: 1-2 drops up to 4 times a day
Non-Steroid Anti-Inflammatory Drugs (NSAIDs)	ketorolac tromethamine (Acular)	≥ 3 years: 1 drop 4 times a day

FIGURE 3-2. OPHTHALMIC ALLERGY MEDICATIONS

- *Antihistamine/Vasoconstrictors.* The use of a combined antihistamine and vasoconstrictor (e.g. *naphazoline + pheniramine*) is more effective than either medication but, as noted above, there is a chance of rebound.
- *Non-Steroid Anti-Inflammatory Drugs (NSAIDs).* Example: *Ketorolac tromethamine* eye drops.
- *Topical steroids.* These are not commonly recommended by allergists, as there may be overlapping microbial infections where steroids may interact adversely.
- *Oral antihistamines.* When allergic conjunctivitis is associated with nasal symptoms (*rhinitis*), then oral antihistamines such as *loratadine*, *fexofenadine* or *cetirizine* alone or in addition to topical eye drops may be effective.

Apart from seasonal and perennial allergic conjunctivitis, there are three other types:

a. *Vernal keratoconjunctivitis*

b. *Atopic keratoconjunctivitis*

c. *Giant papillary conjunctivitis*

VERNAL KERATOCONJUNCTIVITIS (VKC)

VKC is a chronic condition and, as the name implies, it is prevalent in spring (vernal = occurring in spring). Prepubertal boys are more affected than prepubertal girls but the ratio equalizes after puberty. The mean age of onset is 7 years. VKC is more common in warm dry climates, e.g. the Middle East and sub-Saharan Africa. Affected individuals present with bilateral complaints of intense eye itching. The discharge is thick and ropy. Other symptoms include a burning sensation, photophobia, and a foreign body sensation (**Fig. 3-3**).

FIGURE 3-3. CHARACTERISTICS OF VERNAL KERATOCONJUNCTIVITIS	
Symptoms	Bilateral itchy eyes; thick, ropy discharge; burning sensation; photophobia; foreign body sensation
Types	Tarsal or palpebral; limbal; mixed
Sex preference	Boys more common than girls at pre-puberty; normalized ratio after puberty; mean age 7 years
Prevalence	Common in spring; common in warm and dry climates, e.g. Middle East and sub-Saharan Africa

There are three types of VKC: tarsal (palpebral), limbal, and mixed.

In *tarsal (palpebral) VKC*, the affected area is the tarsus (the inside of the eyelid). Giant papillae in the superior tarsus results in a cobblestone appearance. To observe the changes, the upper eyelids should be everted.

In *limbal VKC* the affected area is the limbus (the narrow border between the cornea and sclera). The most affected races are black and Asian. Pathognomonic of the limbal form of conjunctivitis are *Horner-Trantas dots*, which are gelatinous, chalk-white infiltrates of eosinophils and epithelial debris.

In *mixed VKC*, affected individuals have features of both palpebral and limbal forms.

Treatment of Vernal Keratoconjunctivitis

Non-pharmacological Treatment of VKC

In addition to allergen avoidance, cold compresses help. Avoid eye-rubbing, which may worsen the condition.

Pharmacological Treatment of VKC

Managing symptoms of VKC is basically the same as for allergic conjunctivitis. Topical immunomodulators such as *cyclosporine* and *tacrolimus* may also help. However, immunomodulators should be reserved for severe cases or those that do not respond to first line therapy.

Surgical Options

Surgical options such as superficial keratectomy (excision of a portion of cornea) can help to remove plaques and help reepithelialization.

ATOPIC KERATOCONJUNCTIVITIS (AKC)

Patients with chronic AKC are usually atopic; they are frequently asthmatic and may have allergic rhinitis and atopic dermatitis. AKC starts in adulthood, more commonly in males. Affected patients present with bilateral ocular pruritus, lacrimation, blurry vision, photophobia, and a foreign body sensation. The intense eyelid pruritus may result in excoriation (scraped or abraded skin). The patients may suffer from infection with *Staphylococcus aureus* or *Herpes simplex*. Another common finding is punctate epithelial lesions of the cornea and scarring of the cornea and conjunctiva. Affected individuals may also develop cataracts with progression of the disease and the frequent use of topical corticosteroids (**Fig. 3-4**).

FIGURE 3-4. SYMPTOMS OF ATOPIC KERATOCONJUNCTIVITIS	
Symptoms	Bilateral pruritus; lacrimation; blurry vision; photophobia; foreign body sensation
Sex preference	More common in males; onset in adulthood
Visual damage	Excoriation; punctate epithelial lesions of cornea, and scarring affecting cornea and conjunctiva; cataracts
Prevalence	Unknown
Other associated conditions	May be associated with Staphylococcus aureus and Herpes simplex

Treatment of Atopic Keratoconjunctivitis

The treatment of AKC is the same as for VKA. However, the underlying allergic rhinitis and asthma should be identified and treated in affected individuals.

GIANT PAPILLARY CONJUNCTIVITIS (GPC)

GPC is so named because of the finding of large (giant) papillae in the upper tarsal areas. This is not a true allergy but is associated with mechanical irritation from contact lense, ocular sutures, or ocular prostheses and can be exacerbated by ocular allergies. It is more common with soft contact lenses to which allergens can adhere. Affected patients present with ocular pruritus, increased mucus production, superior tarsal hyperemia and protein deposits on contact lenses (whether soft or hard lenses). Some cases may occur with ocular sutures, scleral buckles (used in retinal detachment surgery), filtering blebs (in glaucoma surgery), or eye prostheses (**Fig. 3-5**).

FIGURE 3-5. CHARACTERISTICS OF GIANT PAPILLARY CONJUNCTIVITIS	
Symptoms	Pruritus; redness; increased mucus production
Sex Preference	Either sex
Visual Damage	In chronic condition
Prevalence	Approximately 1-5% of soft contact lens wearers

Treatment of Giant Papillary Conjunctivitis

- Clean contact lenses.
- Avoid wearing contact lenses and rest the eyes for a few weeks.
- Remove other causes, such as exposed sutures.
- Use mast cell stabilizers, antihistamines, and topical steroids if needed.

AUTOIMMUNE DISORDERS AND CONJUNCTIVITIS

Sjogren's syndrome is an autoimmune disorder of the exocrine glands associated with conjunctivitis. The affected patient presents with dry eyes (*keratoconjunctivitis sicca*) and dry mouth (*xerostomia*). There are two types of the Sjogren's syndrome: the *primary* type, which occurs alone, or the *secondary* type, which is associated with other autoimmune disorders such as rheumatoid arthritis, Systemic Lupus Erythematosus (SLE), systemic sclerosis, myasthenia gravis, mixed connective tissue diseases, and primary biliary cirrhosis (**Fig. 3-6**).

Diagnosis of Sjogren's Syndrome

Tear film breakup time (TBUT) tests for ocular dryness. *Flourescein* is placed on the patient's tear film. The patient is asked to blink a few times. The time between the last blink and a dry spot on the tear film is measured. The TBUT < 10 seconds is a sign of evaporation and considered abnormal dryness.

FIGURE 3-6. CONJUNCTIVITIS IN SJOGREN'S SYNDROME	
Symptoms	Dry eyes; dry mouth
Types	Primary; secondary
Sex preference	More in women at or beyond menopause
Visual damage	Epithelial lesion on cornea
Other associated conditions	Rheumatoid arthritis, Systemic Lupus Erythematosus (SLE), systemic sclerosis, myasthenia gravis, mixed connective tissue diseases, or primary biliary cirrhosis

Schirmer's test measures lacrimation. The test is performed by inserting a special filter paper between the lower lid and conjunctiva. Application of an eye anesthetic before the test prevents eye irritation. The patient keeps the eyes closed for 5 minutes. The filter is then removed and the amount of wetting is measured. Wetting < 5 mm indicates reduced tear production.

Treatment of Sjogren's Syndrome

- Patient education. Affected individuals should avoid direct exposure to air-conditioning or heaters.
- Use a humidifier.
- Artificial tears (preferably preservative-free) are the simplest way of managing dry eyes.
- Ointment is useful, especially during sleep.
- Topical cyclosporine (an immunosuppressive).
- Surgically blocking the lacrimal punctum, to prevent tear drainage, requires referral to an ophthalmologist.

CONTACT DERMATITIS OF THE EYES AND EYELIDS

Allergic contact dermatitis of the eyes and eyelids is a type IV Coombs allergic classification (a type of hypersensitivity reaction in which the effector cells, CD4+ T helper and CD8+ T cells are activated by an antigen). This type of allergic reaction is cell-mediated, with delayed manifestations.

The common allergens that affect the eyes and eyelids are cosmetics, eye drop preservatives, and antibiotics. *Thimerosol*, which is used as a preservative in ophthalmic medications, is a potential allergen. Of antibiotics, *neomycin* is known to cause allergic reactions.

Examples of allergens that are directly applied to the eye include eyeliners and eye shadows. Nail polish can cause dermatitis of the eyelids when the eyelids are touched with the fingers.

During history taking, the examiner should get a list of all cosmetics and toiletries the patient uses during the day and night. In addition, investigate whether any of those products are new additions and if the reaction coincides with their time of use.

Management of Contact Dermatitis of the Eyes and Eyelids

- Temporarily avoid all cosmetics to rest the eyes/eyelids and see if this makes a difference.
- Identify and avoid the offending allergen.
- Patch test by an allergist to identify the allergen(s) in question
- Antihistamine eye drops if needed

Chapter 4
Allergic Rhinitis

On exposure to inhalant allergens, susceptible individuals experience a constellation of upper respiratory symptoms, termed *allergic rhinitis*. Although rhinitis literally means nasal inflammation (rhino= nose; itis= inflammation) and the nose is the major affected site, there are other involved areas. An allergic patient may develop nasal symptoms such as nasal congestion, nasal blockage, rhinorrhea (watery nose), nasal pruritus (itching); oral cavity symptoms such as postnasal drip, itchy oral mucosa (especially the palate); sneezing; and plugged ears. The eyes may also become red, watery, and itchy (*allergic conjunctivitis*). Combined "allergic rhinitis" and "allergic conjunctivitis" is called *allergic rhinoconjunctivitis* (**Fig. 4-1**).

FIGURE 4-1. SYMPTOMS OF ALLERGIC RHINITIS AND ALLERGIC RHINOCONJUNCTIVITIS	
ANATOMICAL SITE	**SYMPTOMS**
Eyes	Red, watery, itchy
Nose	Nasal congestion, blocked nose, rhinorrhea (watery nose), itching (mucosa)
Oral cavity	Postnasal drip, itchy oral mucosa (especially palate), sneezing
Ears	Plugged ears

HISTORY AND PHYSICAL EXAM FOR ALLERGIC RHINITIS

Allergic patients are often not familiar with the terms "allergic rhinitis" or "allergic rhinoconjunctivitis"; the examiner should recognize the lay terms for these conditions. The patients may present with complaints of "rose fever" or "hay fever" which are synonymous with "allergic rhinitis."

Although past medical and surgical history, medications, and social history are similar to those of other medical illnesses, there are several pertinent points that specifically should be queried by the examiner:

Symptoms

1. Are your symptoms seasonal? If so, which season is your worst one?

2. Are your symptoms year-round (perennial)?

3. Are your symptoms year-round but worse in a certain season? If so, what season?

Comment: Knowing the length and time of the symptoms helps to narrow the type of allergens. For example if the symptoms occur in summer, the triggers are more likely grass allergens. If the symptoms are year-round, the triggers are more likely indoor allergens.

4. How long have you had the symptoms?

5. Specifically, have you had your symptoms since childhood? Teenage years? Or adulthood?

Comment: Allergic rhinitis usually starts in childhood. Therefore, an elderly patient who presents with complaints of allergy symptoms is likely suffering from *non-allergic rhinitis* (*vasomotor rhinitis*) or rhinitis of other causes.

6. What do you do or have you done to control your symptoms?

Comment: This type of information helps the examiner know the level of treatment needed to manage the patient's condition. The information should reveal the failure and success of medications and help justify termination of a specific medication.

7. How bad are your symptoms? Are they just annoying or are they debilitating? Do you miss school or work days? Do you visit a doctor or an emergency room for flareups?

Comment: This information helps the examiner assess the severity of the symptoms, which is important for formulating disease management.

8. Does the medication control your symptoms?

Comment: The information helps to justify continuing or discontinuing certain medications.

9. What are your symptoms? Red, watery, itchy eyes? Nasal congestion, blocked nose, watery nose, itchy nose? Postnasal drip, itchy mouth and palate, sneezing? Plugged ears?

10. How is your sense of taste and smell?

Comment: Individuals with nasal polyps or chronic sinusitis may have a poor sense of taste or smell.

11. Are you a mouth breather or a nose breather?

Comment: Mouth breathers are likely suffering from nasal blockage.

12. What triggers your symptoms? Pollen, dust, exposure to pets: cat, dog, bird, rabbit, other?

Comment: Information about types of triggers helps the examiner anticipate the type of allergen(s) involved.

History of Medications for Allergic Rhinitis

13. Do you use any over-the-counter nasal sprays or eye drops such as those containing phenylephrine or oxymetazoline?

Comment: Certain medications cause rebound rhinitis, e.g. the nasal decongestant *oxymetazoline*. Repeated use of such decongestants causes a rebound phenomenon termed *rhinitis medicamentosa*. Therefore, it is important to ask about decongestant abuse. Similarly, rebound conjunctivitis can also develop after repeat use of ophthalmic vasoconstrictors.

14. Are you currently taking any antihistamine: oral, nasal, or ophthalmic?
15. If you do not take any antihistamine, is it because of medication failure, side effect, cost, or personal choice?
16. How often do you take your medication(s)? Daily? Just during your season? Is it for a few days at a time or continued throughout the season?

Comment: This information helps the examiner get a feeling for the severity of the patient's symptoms.

Past Medical History for Allergic Rhinitis

17. Do you get sinus infections? If so, how often?

Comment: Patients with allergic rhinitis are prone to sinus infections because the inflammation of nasal passages blocks or partially blocks the passage of mucus secretion, and the stagnant mucus may become infected. Abnormal nasal anatomy, such as after a nasal fracture, may also explain frequent sinusitis. Finally, frequent sinus infections (more than 5-6/year) may be a clue to underlying humoral immunodeficiency (specifically IgG).

18. Have you ever had pneumonia? Frequently (more than 4-5 times/year)?

Comment: Frequent pneumonia is a clue to possible underlying humoral immunodeficiency (specifically reduced IgG). In children, frequent otitis media may also be a clue to humoral immunodeficiency.

19. Do you have asthma?

Comment: Some patients suffer from asthma while others have "respiratory allergy." In respiratory allergy, the lung function is normal but the patient expresses asthma-like symptoms such as shortness of breath, chest tightness, or wheezing upon exposure to an inhalant allergen (see **Chapter 8**).

Past Surgical History

20. Have you had nasal surgery? If so, what type? Nasal fracture, turbinoplasty (reduction of nasal turbinate bones)? Septoplasty (correction of deviated septum)? Polypectomy (removal of nasal polyps)?

Comment: The type of surgery helps the examiner better understand the pathology of the nasal problem and its relationship to the rhinitis.

22. Have you had any operation on your ears, such as ear tubes?

Comment: The cause of repeated ear tube placements in children needs to be investigated, as it may be a clue to underlying humoral immunodeficiency (specifically IgG deficiency).

Family History

23. Do any of your immediate family (parents, siblings or children) have allergic rhinitis, asthma, food allergy, drug allergy, latex allergy, eczema, or immunodeficiency?

Environmental History

It is important to get a through history of the patient's work and home environment. Such information helps the clinician better understand the type and level of exposure to allergens and irritants.

Home Environment

24. Where do you live? In town, downtown, in mountains, close to freeway?

Comment: The habitat relates to the type of exposure to allergens and irritants. For example, living close to a Freeway makes the individual vulnerable to exhaust fumes and pollution from passing vehicles. The danger of such exposures has been noted and documented in asthmatic patients. Those who live in the mountains may have more exposure to pollens.

25. What kind of building do you live in? House, apartment, duplex?
26. How old is the building?

Comment: An older home may have problems with plumbing, such as leakage that can increase humidity. Humidity over 50% is a suitable environment for mold growth, dust mites and cockroach infestation.

27. How many levels is your residence? Is it a single floor?

Comment: This is important to know as it relates to the air circulation system. For example, a two-story building may share the same HVAC (heating, ventilating, and air conditioning) system, and if there are pollutants or airborne allergens they may spread from one floor to another.

28. Do you have a basement? If you do, is it damp? Does it flood with rain? Do you live in the basement?

Comment: A damp basement is ideal for mold growth.

29. What type of heater do you use at home? Central, furnace, or fireplace?
30. What type of cooling system do you use? Central, window unit, or fan?

Comment: A contaminated heating, ventilation, and air conditioning (HVAC) system is a source of distribution of indoor allergens, microorganisms, mold spores, and bacterial toxins. Therefore, it is crucial to inquire about the source of HVAC used and its condition. For example, an improper setting of HVAC can set the stage for increasing humidity and mold growth or survival of dust mites. Also, infrequent changing of air filters, and water leakage in an air-conditioning unit can cause bacterial growth and room air contamination.

31. Do you have windows? Are they sealed or can they be opened? How often do you open your windows?

Comment: Mold spores, pollen, and other inhalant allergens can enter the indoor environment through an open door or a window; therefore, this type of information is important when investigating the level of allergen exposure.

32. What type of flooring do you have? Carpet, tile, hardwood, or linoleum?

Comment: Dust mites like to settle in carpet. Information about flooring helps understand the level of dust mite distribution and exposure.

33. What type of bedding do you have? Mattress only (near the floor)? Mattress over a box spring?
34. What material comprises your blanket, pillow, or mattress? Feathers or synthetics?

Comment: Dust mites survive by ingesting organic matter such as human skin or feathers.

35. What type of furniture do you have? Leather, vinyl, wooden, upholstered?

Comment: Although dust mites settle on all types of furniture; they settle deeply in layers of upholstered furniture, making it a cleaning challenge. Also inquire about other types of furniture such as bookshelves, as they are also a source of accumulation for dust mites.

36. Do you have an aquarium?

Comment: Aquariums may sustain mold growth.

37. Do you have pets? If so, are they indoor or outdoor pets? Do they come into your bedroom? Do you sleep with your pet at night?

Work Environment

38. What is your working environment? Office building? Classroom? Warehouse? Outdoors (letter carrier, peace officer, firefighter, gardener)?

Comment: Unlike residential buildings, newer commercial buildings commonly have sealed windows, which eliminates the chance of direct entry of pollen into the indoor environment.

39. How many employees work in the same room?

Comment: The more employees in the same area, the more furniture used and more airborne allergens. For example, if there are more employees in a single room, there would be more cubicles. Most cubicles are padded with fabrics that accumulate dust mites. In addition, the more employees in a room, the higher chance they carry allergens with them (e.g. cat or dog dander on their clothing). Also, the more employees in a single room, the higher chance of exposure to fumes such as perfumes that may cause respiratory irritation in susceptible individuals.

40. Do co-workers bring pets to work?

Comment: In some jobs, employees are allowed to bring their pets to work. In other situations, co-workers may carry dog or cat dander on their clothing. Direct exposure to pets or pet dander can trigger allergy symptoms.

Occupational History

The patient's occupational history is important. Some professions make susceptible individuals more vulnerable to allergic reactions. A list of such professions and the type of allergies are summarized in **Figure 4-2**.

FIGURE 4-2. PROFESSIONALS SUSCEPTIBLE TO ALLERGIES		
PROFESSION	**EXPOSURE**	**TYPE OF ALLERGIES**
Landscaper/gardener/ forest ranger	Pollens	Allergic rhinitis; insect allergy
Painter	Pollens; insects	Allergic rhinitis; insect allergy
Veterinarian	Animal dander: cat, dog, etc	Allergic rhinitis; asthma; allergic contact dermatitis
Pet store employee	Animal dander: cat, dog, etc	Allergic rhinitis; asthma; allergic contact dermatitis
Pet groomer	Animal dander: cat, dog, etc	Allergic rhinitis; asthma; allergic contact dermatitis

Review of Systems

Specific key information:

HEENT: Glasses, red eyes, nasal polyps, ear tubes, recurrent ear infections

Heart: Palpitations (Note: this may be a side effect of certain medications such as albuterol, a bronchodilator)

Lungs: Shortness of breath, wheezing, chest tightness, cough

Genitourinary (GU): Urinary retention, a potential side effect of oral decongestants such as pseudoephedrine

Skin: Eczema. This is a clue to a history of atopy (genetic predisposition to allergies)

Ob/Gyn: Rhinitis may occur during pregnancy.

PHYSICAL EXAMINATION

HEENT:

Eyes: Check for conjunctivitis.

Shiner (black eye): A darkened discoloration under the eyes commonly seen in allergic patients. This is likely due to obstruction or impeded venous blood flow due to nasal congestion.

Ears: Look for erythema, ear tubes, pus.

Nose: Nasal crease. This is a horizontal crease on the lower bridge of the nose, formed after repeatedly rubbing the nose upward with the palm of the hand as a reaction to nasal itching. There may also be rhinitis, enlarged turbinates, nasal polyps (non-cancerous tissue growths in the nasal passage or sinuses). Depending on the location, polyps may be seen by the naked eye or with an otoscope. Nasal endoscopy can help to visualize more distal polyps.

Oral: Erythema, postnasal drip

HEART: Tachycardia (side effect of some medications such as albuterol)

LUNGS: Poor ventilation, wheezing, rhonchi

SKIN: Eczema, hives, angioedema

No other exam unless a specific abnormality warrants further investigation.

TREATMENT OF ALLERGIC RHINITIS

The treatment of allergic rhinitis involves:

- Avoidance of allergens
- Environmental control
- Short-term treatment
- Long-term treatment

Avoidance

The best strategy to fight allergies in general is avoidance. Sometimes a few simple steps are all that is needed to achieve control of allergy symptoms. For example, the allergic patient should avoid going outdoors on windy days with high pollen counts. Brightly colored shirts with printed flowers attract bees. Perfumes and scented toiletry can also attract insects, such as yellow jackets. Extra precaution in wearing suitable clothing and in using toiletry is a big step toward avoiding bee stings.

Environmental Control (Fig. 4-3)

We have no control of the outdoor environment except avoiding extreme weather. However, we can implement a few measures to control the indoor environment:

1. Close the windows on days with high pollen counts. Some commercial buildings have sealed windows, which helps stop outdoor allergens from entering indoors.

2. Keep the building humidity below 55%. High humidity favors the growth of molds and survival of dust mites and cockroaches.

FIGURE 4-3. ENVIRONMENTAL CONTROL OF ALLERGIES		
	TYPE OF PRECAUTION	**OTHER RECOMMENDATIONS**
Outdoor Allergens: Pollens	• Avoid going outdoors on days with high pollen counts. • Avoid mowing lawn. • Close windows on windy days and days with high pollen counts. • Avoid bringing outdoor allergens indoors.	• Check pollen counts from local designated station in your community. • If you have to mow the lawn, wear a face mask and shower and change clothing after done. • After playing outdoors on grass, children need to shower and change clothing before going to bed.
Insects	• Do not use perfumes when camping outdoors or on a picnic. • Avoid attracting insects.	• Use unscented toiletry. • Wear clothing without flower prints or bright colors.
Indoor Allergens	• Control indoor humidity. • Do not attract cockroaches to the kitchen. • Keep pet danders out of the bedroom. • Clean the dust on flat surfaces regularly. • Do not use upholstered furniture. • Avoid using feather pillows, comforters and beddings. • Cover bedding to avoid penetration of dust mites. • Do not use carpet on floors, especially in bedrooms and living room.	• Keep the indoor humidity below 55%. • Keep the kitchen clean; trash containers closed. • Keep pets out of bedroom and close the bedroom vents. • Wipe bookshelves, tables, and furniture regularly with a damp cloth. • Use leather, vinyl, or non-upholstered furniture for easy cleaning. • Use a synthetic (non-organic) pillow, comforter, or bedding. • Encase mattress, box springs and pillow with dust mite-proof material. • Use hardwood or tile flooring in bedroom and living room.

3. Dust indoor areas regularly to prevent accumulation of dust on furniture, bookshelves, and flat-surface areas such as countertops and tables.

4. Use non-feather pillows and comforters; dust mites live and survive in organic matter.

5. Wash bed sheets in hot water once every week or two to help destroy and wash out dust mites. Human skin sheds about a couple of grams of dead skin in 24 hours; this is enough food for dust mites to survive and propagate.

6. Envelope mattresses, box springs, and pillowcases with dust mite-proof encasing to prevent dust mite entry.

7. Use hardwood or tile floors. Dust mites enter the deeper portions of carpets, which makes their elimination a challenge.

Short-Term Treatment of Allergic Rhinitis

The short-term treatment of allergic rhinitis is temporary relief of allergic symptoms with medication; this is advantageous to those whose symptoms last only a few weeks a year. A disadvantage of short-term treatment is *tachyphylaxis,* a rapid decrease in response to a medication after repeated use.

Medications for Allergic Rhinitis (Fig. 4-4)

FIGURE 4-4. MEDICATIONS FOR ALLERGIC RHINITIS		
CLASS	**FORMS OF DELIVERY**	**EXAMPLE(S)**
Antihistamines	Nasal	azelastine; olopatadine
	Ophthalmic	emedastine
	Oral	• First generation: diphenhydramine • Second generation: loratadine; fexofenadine; cetirizine
Mast cell stabilizers	Ophthalmic	pemirolast; cromolyn sodium
Antihistamine-mast cell stabilizers	Ophthalmic	azelastine; olopatadine
Sympathomimetics	Ophthalmic	naphazoline
	Nasal	oxymetazoline
	Oral	pseudoephedrine
Antihistamine-sympathomimetics	Oral	loratadine-D; fexofenadine-D; cetirizine-D
Non-steroid anti-inflammatory drugs (NSAIDs)	Ophthalmic	ketorolac
Leukotriene receptor antagonists	Oral	montelukast; zafirlukast
Glucocorticoids	Nasal	fluticasone; triamcinolone acetonide
	Oral	prednisone

1. ***Antihistamines.*** The leading class of medication for allergic symptom control is antihistamines. This class of medication acts by blocking histamine H1 receptors and reducing/stopping the symptoms. The older generation antihistamines such as diphenhydramine have cholinergic side effects such as dry mouth and sedation, because they pass through the blood-brain barrier.

   The newer generation antihistamines, such as *loratadine* and *fexofenadine*, have minimal or no sedative side effect. The antihistamines are marketed in oral, nasal, and ophthalmic forms. When the allergic symptoms are localized to the nose or eyes, nasal sprays or topical ophthalmics are preferred. If the symptoms involve more than one system, such as oral, nasal, ocular, and respiratory, then the oral form of antihistamine is recommended.

2. ***Mast cell stabilizers*** are an alternative method of preventing allergic symptoms. Stabilizing mast cells prevents their degranulation, which in turn prevents histamine release.

   Some medications, such as *azelastine ophthalmic* work as both antihistamine and mast cell stabilizers.

3. ***Sympathomimetics*** are decongestants, which are marketed as a single drug (e.g. *pseudoephedrine*) or in combination with antihistamines such as *loratadine-D* (loratadine and pseudoephedrine). These drugs are also marketed in nasal form, for decongestion, and in ophthalmic form.

4. ***Non-Steroid Anti-Inflammatory Drugs (NSAIDs).*** This class of medication in ophthalmic form is used to relieve pruritus due to ocular allergy.

5. ***Leukotriene receptor antagonists.*** Leukotrienes, products of arachidonic acid, are released from many different cells, including mast cells and eosinophils. They cause inflammation of the airways and smooth muscle contraction. Blocking the leukotriene receptors results in an anti-inflammatory effect and bronchodilation in asthmatics. Since leukotrienes are also released in nasal mucosa, leukotriene receptor antagonists help control allergic rhinitis symptoms.

6. ***Glucocorticoids.*** This class of medication is used in nasal sprays and ophthalmic and oral preparations. The recommendation for using the ophthalmic form is reserved for the ophthalmologist, as glucocorticoids may have an adverse effect in certain ocular infections. The use of oral glucocorticoids in controlling symptoms of allergic rhinitis is uncommon.

Long-Term Treatment of Allergic Rhinitis

Preventive environmental measures and medications are temporary, short-term treatments for allergic rhinitis. When these measures fail, the long-term therapy is *immunomodulation* (alteration of the immune system) with the use of *immunotherapy*, a treatment regimen that renders an allergic patient immune to the harm of a specific allergen (see **Chapter 11**).

Chapter 5
Urticaria and Angioedema

Urticaria (from Latin *urtica*: nettle), also known as *hives*, is an erythematous, raised, and pruritic area of the skin that results from release of histamine by mast cells or basophils. Urticaria can present locally in the area of contact with an allergen (*contact urticaria*) or generalized across the skin.

Angioedema is an edematous area of skin that results from release of histamine by mast cells or basophils. It affects loose connective tissues, as in the face, lips, larynx, genitalia or extremities. Angioedema may or may not be associated with urticaria.

The similarities and differences of urticaria and angioedema are summarized in **Figure 5-1**.

FIGURE 5-1. CHARACTERISTICS OF URTICARIA AND ANGIOEDEMA		
	URTICARIA	**ANGIOEDEMA**
Location	Superficial layer of dermis	Deeper layer of dermis
Distribution	Usually neck, torso, extremities	Lips, eyelids, periorbital area, tongue, larynx, pharynx, extremities, genitalia, smooth muscle lining of the gut
Symptoms	Pruritus	Burning sensation

PATHOPHYSIOLOGY OF URTICARIA AND ANGIOEDEMA

The pathophysiology of urticaria and angioedema involves degranulation of mast cells. The cascade of events starts by binding a specific IgE to the high affinity receptor FceRI on the mast cell surface. Then the mast cells become activated and release various chemicals, including histamine, in a process called *degranulation* (**Fig. 2-6**).

Mast cell degranulation may also be a non-IgE-mediated phenomenon. An example is the direct effect of vancomycin or polymixin B on mast cells. But there is another mechanism, *Gell-Coombs Type III hypersensitivity* (e.g. serum sickness), involving damage done by antibody/antigen complexes, which can cause urticaria.

The major inflammatory mediator released in mast cell degranulation is histamine, which causes a wheal and flare. In the *triple reaction of Lewis,* there are, after stroking the skin, *erythema* (an initial red line), a result of capillary dilatation; then a reddish *flare* around the line, a result of arteriolar dilatation; and, finally, a *wheal,* which is extravasation of fluid due to vascular permeability (**Fig. 5-2**).

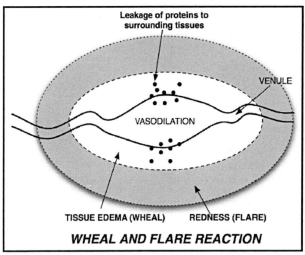

FIGURE 5-2. (From Mahmoudi, M. Immunology Made Ridiculously Simple, Medmaster)

The difference in presentation of symptoms in urticaria and angioedema has to do with the affected location within the skin. Urticaria occurs in the superficial layer of dermis whereas angioedema occurs in deeper layers. Both skin conditions are consequences of the release of histamines from mast cells and basophils (**Plate 5-1**).

CLASSIFICATION

Urticaria and angioedema are either acute, defined by reactions lasting less than 6-8 weeks, or chronic, which are reactions lasting more than 8 weeks.

Fifty percent of affected individuals have urticaria alone, 40% have urticaria and angioedema, and 10% have angioedema alone (**Fig. 5-3**).

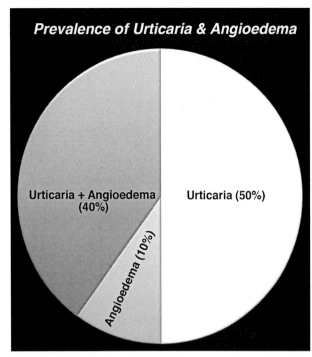

FIGURE 5-3.

ETIOLOGY

The causes of urticaria and angioedema, summarized in **Figure 5-4**, are as follows:

FIGURE 5-4. CAUSES OF URTICARIA AND ANGIOEDEMA
Food allergy
Inhalent allergens
Drugs
Dermographism
Cold-induced
Heat-induced
Solar-induced
Aquatic
Pressure-induced
Vibration-induced angioedema
Exercise-induced urticaria
Insect stings/bites
Contact with allergen
Hereditary angioedema (HAE)
Acquired angioedema
Idiopathic

Food Allergy. Although any food can potentially cause urticaria and/or angioedema, the common allergenic foods are milk, soy, eggs, wheat, nuts, peanuts, fish, and shellfish (**Fig. 5-5**). Food additives such as *tartrazine* (a yellow azo dye) are also a potential cause of urticaria/angioedema.

FIGURE 5-5. COMMON FOOD ALLERGENS	
TYPE	**EXAMPLES**
Dairy	Milk, eggs
Protein	Soy
Grains	Wheat
Nuts	Almonds, walnuts, pistachios
Legumes	Peanuts
Fish	Halibut, cod
Shellfish	Shrimp, oyster, crab

Inhalent Allergens. Certain susceptible individuals may develop urticaria upon contact with dogs or cats. Therefore, allergy testing of such individuals for inhalants is warranted.

Drugs. Many drugs can potentially induce urticaria/angioedema. However, the two most common ones are non-steroid anti-inflammatory drugs (NSAIDs) and angiotensin-converting enzyme (ACE) inhibitors. Others include vaccines, such as allergen extracts used in immunotherapy. As will be discussed in detail in **Chapter 11**, allergy immunotherapy entails injection of increasing doses of an allergen extract. At a certain dose, depending on the body's immune response, the reaction to the allergen manifests as an urticaria, a red pruritic welt. Some examples of drugs that induce allergic reactions are listed in **Figure 5-6**.

FIGURE 5-6. EXAMPLES OF DRUG-INDUCED URTICARIA/ANGIOEDEMA	
CLASS	**EXAMPLE(S)**
Antibiotics	Penicillin, sulfa
Cyclooxygenase inhibitors	Aspirin, NSAIDs
Antihypertensive medications	Angiotensin-converting enzyme inhibitors, diuretics, beta blockers
Enzymes	Papain (found in papaya; used as a meat tenderizer and to process beer)
Hormones	Birth control pills
Vaccines	Allergen extracts
Others	Drugs containing yellow dye (angioedema)

Physical urticaria is induced with a variety of physical activities: *Dermographism* (or *Dermatographism*) is a type of physical urticaria that results after stroking the skin with a blunt object (**Plate 5-2**). *Cold-induced urticaria* is induced by exposure to a cold environment such as cold weather, cold water, or a cold object, e.g. holding a cold steering wheel of a car in winter. The reaction of a susceptible individual to cold may manifest as a contact urticaria, such as holding a cold object, or may be systemic, such as anaphylaxis after jumping into a cold swimming pool.

There are several types of cold-induced urticaria (**Fig. 5-7**)

FIGURE 5-7. TYPES OF COLD-INDUCED URTICARIA	
TYPE	**COMMENT**
Primary Cold Urticaria	Also known as Primary Urticaria
Secondary Cold Urticaria	Associated with systemic disease
Cold Reflex Urticaria	Occurs in the adjacent area of cold exposure
Cold-Induced Cholinergic Urticaria	Occurs in the presence of cold and exercise; small in size
Cold-Induced Dermographism	Occurs after stroking the skin with a cold object

- *Primary (or idiopathic) cold urticaria* is a type of urticaria with an unidentified cause.

- *Secondary cold urticaria* is a type of cold urticaria that is associated with systemic diseases, including cryoglobulinemia, cryofibrinogenemia, and leukoclastic vasculitis. Sometimes this type of urticaria is associated with infectious diseases such as syphilis, rubeola, or parasitic infections.

- *Cold reflex urticaria* develops in skin areas adjacent to the cold-exposed area.

- *Cold-induced cholinergic urticaria* depends on the existence of two factors: cold environment and exercise. The morphology of this type of urticaria is smaller than typical urticaria.

- *Cold-dependent dermographism* develops after stroking the skin with a chilled object.

Heat-induced urticaria is caused by exposure to heat; the heat source may be hot water or a hot ambiance such as a hot room or a hot object. The reaction may be just local, as by holding a hot object in the hand, or systemic such as anaphylaxis after jumping into an overheated jacuzzi.

Solar-induced urticaria is induced by exposure to sunlight. Interestingly, susceptible individuals react to a specific range of wavelength. Most studies report that wavelengths of 300-500 nm elicit the urticarial response (**Fig. 5-8**). The typical symptoms are itching and burning; however headaches, dizziness, wheezing and, rarely, anaphylaxis may occur.

Aquatic urticaria is a rare form of urticaria that results after exposure to water, regardless of water temperature.

FIGURE 5-8. TYPES OF SOLAR-INDUCED URTICARIA	
TYPE OF LIGHT	**RANGE OF WAVELENGTH Å (ANGSTROM)**
Visible	380-700
UVA (ultraviolet-A)	320-400
UVB (ultraviolet-B)	280-320
Infrared (rare)	Above 700

Pressure-induced urticaria results after prolonged pressure. One type develops under the straps of a heavy backpack after several hours of continuous contact.

Vibration-induced angioedema occurs after a few minutes of vibration, e.g. after using a jackhammer.

Exercise-induced urticaria results from exercise, such as running or playing a variety of sports. Affected individuals may even experience anaphylaxis (*exercise-induced anaphylaxis*).

Insect stings or bites can cause urticaria and/or angioedema. For example, if a yellow jacket stings an extremity you may have urticaria or angioedema but if it stings the eyelids, lips, or tongue, you would have angioedema. Some other examples of insects that may cause urticaria/angioedema are fire ants and "kissing bugs."

Vasculitis is a type of allergy (Coombs Type III) in which an antigen-antibody complex precipitates in blood vessels. An urticarial hive spot should last less than 24 hours. If it lasts longer than 24 hours, you should suspect vasculitis. *Serum sickness* is an example of vasculitis that manifests after 10-14 days of taking medications such as an antibiotic, or antiserum.

Urticaria pigmentosa is the most common skin manifestation of systemic *mastocytosis*, a disease characterized by an abnormal increase in the number of mast cells. Patches of darkened skin are often seen, along with intense itching.

Infection should be considered a part of the workup of underlying urticaria. Some infections such as hepatitis B may cause urticaria.

Malignancies associated with urticaria include lymphoma and myeloproliferative disorders.

Contact with allergen. A susceptible individual may develop urticaria upon contact with a chemical substance or a biological agent. A common example is contact with latex gloves by health care providers. Other examples include skin exposure to animals, food (e.g. after peeling an apple), or drugs.

Hereditary angioedema, acquired angioedemas, and angioedema without urticaria. *Hereditary angioedema (HAE)* is an autosomal dominant disorder that develops as a result of deficiency of an enzyme, C1 esterase inhibitor (C1-inh). This enzyme normally binds to and inhibits C1, the first complement of the complement system (**Fig. 2-9**). Complement is a group of proteins, mostly enzyme precursors, that are found in the serum and, when activated, undergo cascading reactions that promote inflammation, lysis of bacteria and enhanced removal of antigen- antibody complexes.

Without C1-inh, C1 becomes overactive, leading to an increase in the inflammatory response. In addition, C1-inh normally inhibits kinin production. Low or dysfunctional C1-inh enzyme results in accumulation of bradykinin, leading to increased vascular permeability and angioedema.

There are three types of HAE: *Type 1 (HAE1), Type 2 (HAE2)*, and *Type 3 (HAE3)*. HAE1 comprises the majority (85%) of HAE. In this type of HAE, the C1-inh level is low. In HAE2, the level of C1-inh is normal but the enzyme that inhibits C1-inh is overreactive. HAE3 is a rare type of HAE characterized by normal serum C4 and C1-inh protein as well as normal C1-inh activity (**Fig. 5-9**).

Acquired angioedema may be secondary to lymphoma, to autoantibodies against C1-inh or immune complex mediated depletion of C1-inh.

Angioedema without urticaria: Angioedema without urticaria is either hereditary or acquired.

C3b/C4b inactivator deficiency. C3b/C4b inactivator (complement Factor I) is one of the regulatory proteins of the complement system which, in the presence of other regulatory factors, cleaves C3b and C4b into several fragments that do not participate in complement activation (**Fig. 2-9**). *C3b/C4b inactivator deficiency* is a rare hereditary cause of urticaria and angioedema. Lack of this enzyme results in activation of complement.

DIAGNOSIS OF URTICARIA AND ANGIOEDEMA

Dermographism. To test for dermographism, you can take a blunt object such as a key and stroke the volar aspect of the forearm. The appearance of a red raised area in about 5 minutes indicates a positive reaction. The shape of the resulting urticaria depends on the type of object used. If the stroke is linear, then the urticaria appears as a linear area (*linear hives*).

Prick Skin Test. The *prick skin test* is used to identify the specific antibody to inhalant or food.

Cold-induced Urticaria. The *ice cube test* can diagnose cold-induced urticaria. An ice cube is placed on a volar aspect of a forearm for 5 minutes. A hive with the size of the exposed ice cube surface appears under the ice-exposed area.

Heat-induced Urticaria. A positive test results after a hot bath or exercise.

Solar-induced Urticaria. Phototesting is utilized to determine the spectrum of the light as well as the *minimum urticarial dose* (*MUD*) that can elicit the urticaria. The test simply entails the exposure of the test subject to different doses of various light sources and observing the reactions.

Pressure-Induced Urticaria. The application of a 15 lb pressure for 15 minutes suffices to demonstrate pressure-induced urticaria. One way to do this is to wear a backpack for 15 minutes. Susceptible individuals will develop urticaria under the shoulder straps.

Vibratory Angioedema. The test can be performed by placing the arm on a vibratory machine, such as a Vortex, for few minutes and observing the vibrated area for urticaria.

Contact Urticaria. A simple way to test for this urticaria is direct contact with the suspected allergen. The *Use Test* consists of wearing latex gloves for a few minutes and checking for urticaria in the area of contact.

Hereditary and Acquired Angioedema. The workup should include measuring serum C1, C2, C4, C1-inh level and C1-inh functional level. However, measuring C4 suffices for the initial diagnosis of hereditary angioedema.

Urticaria Pigmentosa. Skin biopsy.

C3b Inactivator Deficiency. Test for C3, factor B, C3b inactivator.

Figure 5-10 summarizes the diagnostic tests for urticaria and angioedema.

FIGURE 5-9. TYPES OF ANGIOEDEMA					
CHARACTERISTICS	**HAE1**	**HAE2**	**HAE3**	**ACQUIRED**	**HISTAMINE-INDUCED**
Bradykinin induced	+	+	+	+	−
Histamine induced	−	−	−	−	+
IgE-mediated	−	−	−	−	+ or −
Prevalence	85%	15%	Rare	Rare	High
C4	Low	Normal	Normal	Low	Not affected
C1-inh	Low	Normal	Normal	Low	Not affected
C1-inh activity	Low	Low	Normal	Low	Not affected

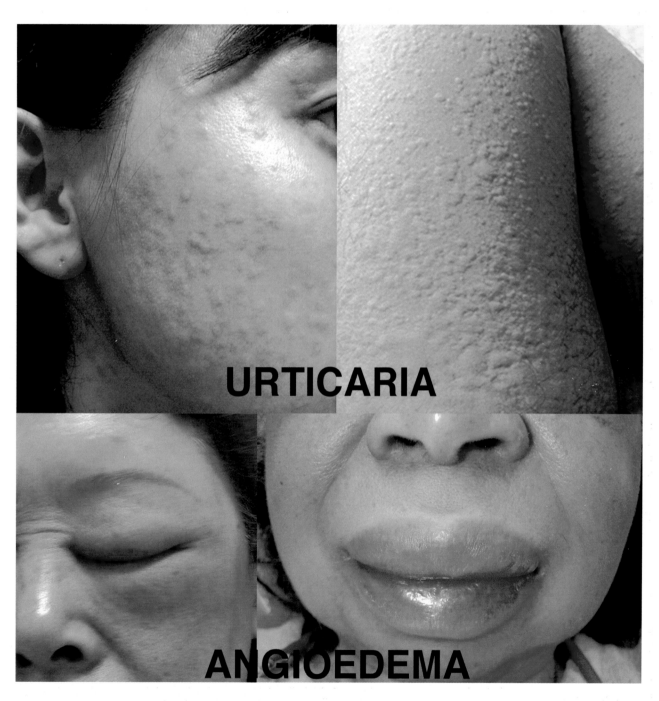

Plate 5-1. Urticaria and angioedema. (Courtesy of Professor Satoshi Yoshida)

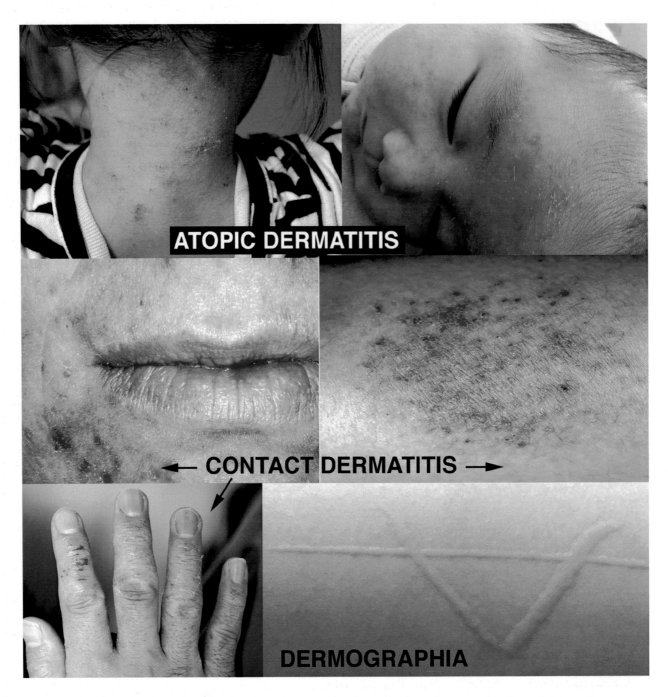

Plate 5-2. Atopic dermatitis, contact dermatitis, and dermographia. (Courtesy of Professor Satoshi Yoshida)

FIGURE 5-10. DIAGNOSTIC TESTS FOR URTICARIA AND ANGIOEDEMA

CAUSE	TEST
Dermographism	Stroke the ventral aspect of a forearm and wait for 5 minutes for reaction.
Food allergy	Prick skin test (a specific IgE response).
Inhalent allergy	Prick skin test (a specific IgE response).
Cold-induced urticaria	Ice cube test: apply an ice cube to the volar aspect of an arm for 5 minutes.
Heat-induced urticaria	Exposure to warm water
Solar-induced urticaria	Exposure to various light sources with different wavelengths
Pressure-induced urticaria	Apply 15 lbs pressure for 15 minutes on the test area.
Vibratory angioedema	Apply vibration on the test area, such as placing a hand on a Vortex for 4 minutes.
Contact urticaria	Exposure (contact) with the allergen. Example: the " Use Test" for latex allergy by wearing latex gloves for few minutes.
Hereditary angioedema	C1, C2, C4, C1-inh, C1-inh functional assay
Urticaria pigmentosa	Skin biopsy
C3b Inactivator deficiency	C3, factor B, C3b inactivator

PREVENTION AND TREATMENT OF URTICARIA AND ANGIOEDEMA

Prevention

The best way to prevent urticaria and angioedema is to identify and avoid the suspected trigger. For example, if heat or cold is the trigger, then focus on avoiding the extreme temperature. Unless the reaction is life-threatening (e.g. laryngioedema or anaphylaxis), one can just limit future exposure to the trigger. Examples include limited time spent for showering in hot water in those with heat-induce urticaria or limited exposure to water in those with aquatic urticaria.

Medications for Urticaria and Angioedema

1. **Antihistamines** can be used to alleviate the pruritus and discomfort and to reduce the reaction. Topical antihistamines may be used for a small local reaction while an oral form is recommended for general reactions. A quickly dissolving form of antihistamines such as *diphenhydramine disintegrating strips* is a superior form of antihistamine for those with laryngioedema. This is because the medication bypasses the conventional oral route of ingestion; its absorption in the mouth takes a few short seconds.

2. **Corticosteroids**, either topical (cream/ointment) or oral, may alleviate the inflammation and control pruritus.

3. **Anti-IgE Antibody.** More recently, *omalizumab*, an anti-IgE antibody, has been approved for management of chronic urticaria.

The prevention and treatment of urticaria and angioedema are summarized in **Figure 5-11**.

FIGURE 5-11. PREVENTION AND TREATMENT OF URTICARIA AND ANGIOEDEMA

STRATEGY	COMMENT	EXAMPLES
Prevention: Reduce exposure	Avoid the trigger	Avoid extreme hot and cold temperature or the offending medication.
	Avoid extended exposure to the trigger	Decrease showering/ bathing time in extreme temperature in heat- or cold-induced urticaria.
Medication	Topical cream for local reaction	Topical antihistamines or corticosteroids
	Oral antihistamine: H1 blocker H2 blocker H1 and H2 blocker	Oral antihistamines for general reactions, such as *diphenhydramine* or *cetirizine* (H1 blockers)
		Ranitidine (H2 blocker)
		Doxepin (tricyclic antidepressant), a potent H1 and H2 blocker
	Oral steroids	*Prednisone* or *methylprednisolone*
	Anti-IgE antibody	Injectable medication for chronic urticaria
	Other anti-inflammatory drugs	Cyclosporine
	C1-inh replacement	Plasma-derived or recombinant C1-inh for treatment of hereditary angioedema
	Kallikrein blocker	*Ecallantide* for treatment of hereditary angioedema
	Bradykinin antagonist	*Icatibant* for treatment of hereditary angioedema

Chapter 6
Atopic Dermatitis

Atopic dermatitis (AD) is a chronic relapsing inflammatory skin condition. It is a complicated disease that is genetically transmitted. Affected patients show high levels of peripheral IgE.

AD is more prevalent in infants and children, but it is also seen in adults. Affected individuals commonly have other types of allergies, such as allergic rhinitis or asthma.

DIAGNOSIS OF ATOPIC DERMATITIS

Atopic dermatitis is a clinical diagnosis. It has several diagnostic classifications, but the simplest way of diagnosing AD is the presence of the triad of atopy (hereditary predisposition), eczematous lesions (erythematous, scaly and vesicular areas) and pruritus (**Fig. 6-1**).

FIGURE 6-1. CLINICAL FEATURES OF ATOPIC DERMATITIS	
FEATURE	**NOTE**
Pruritus	Usually leads to excoriations of skin lesions
Skin involvement (eczema)	See Figure 6-3
Past history of allergies or family history of allergies in first-degree relatives	Examples: allergic rhinitis; asthma
Relapsing skin lesions	Due to exposure to irritants/ triggers

The area of skin involvement differs in infants and adults. In infants and younger children, the common areas are face, neck, and extensor surfaces. The diaper area is usually spared. In older children and adults, the distribution changes from extensor to flexor surfaces of the limbs (**Figs. 6-2** and **Plate 5-2**).

While basically a disease of infancy and childhood, atopic dermatitis may continue into adolescence and adulthood. New onset of the disease in adulthood, although possible, is rare. AD commonly starts between 3 to 6 months of age. Most patients develop it in the first year of life and 90% by age 5. In general, AD affects 10 to 20% of children and 1 to 3% of adults.

FIGURE 6-2. DISTRIBUTION OF ATOPIC DERMATITIS RASH		
AGE GROUP	**AREAS OF SKIN INVOLVEMENT**	**NOTE**
Infants	Scalp, face, neck, trunk, *extensor* surfaces of the limbs	Diaper area is usually spared
Older children	*Flexor* surfaces of the limbs, neck, wrists, ankle, infragluteal area	Other areas may also be involved
Adults	*Flexor* surfaces, neck, face	Other areas may also be involved

RISK FACTORS FOR ATOPIC DERMATITIS

Atopy, being a genetic predisposition to allergies, is an important risk factor for developing AD. A mutation in the *FLG gene* has been recognized as a risk factor. The FLG gene normally encodes *profilaggrin*, which breaks down to *filaggrin*, which contributes to skin epidermal hydration. Decrease in filagarin results in dry skin, as in atopic dermatitis.

TRIGGERS OF ATOPIC DERMATITIS

Physical factors such as irritants and emotional factors can trigger AD and cause flareups. These triggers differ from one individual to another. One should attempt to identify the sources of the flareup and avoid them. Physical triggers include sweating as a result of hot and humid weather or physical activity, such as exercise that increases body temperature and perspiration. An AD flareup may also be due to direct contact with certain detergents and chemicals. For example, some patients' symptoms may worsen with certain soaps or laundry or cleaning detergents (**Fig. 6-3**). Food allergy is an important trigger in at least 33% of children. Food hypersensitivity can be detected by skin prick testing and serum IgE testing; however, due to the high percentage of false positive reactions, the results should be interpreted with caution.

FIGURE 6-3. TRIGGERS OF ATOPIC DERMATITIS	
TRIGGER	**COMMENTS**
Weather	Hot and humid weather can result in sweating and flare. Cold weather can dry the skin, which worsens the skin rash of the affected patients.
Physical activity	Skin flare-up after exercise and sweating
Food	Certain foods may trigger AD, e.g. spicy foods.
Dry skin	Frequent hand washing not only irritates skin, but also results in dry skin, causing flareups of eczema.
Chemicals	Soaps, detergents and other chemicals that come in contact with the skin can potentially exacerbate the eczema.
Allergens	Pollens, molds, dust mites, food (e.g. milk, eggs, and soy in children)
Cosmetics	
Perfumes	
Cigarette smoke	
Infectious agents	With a break in the skin barrier, infectious agents can pass through the epidermis and cause infections, hence exacerbating the eczema.
Emotional factors	E.g. stress, anger

DIFFERENTIAL DIAGNOSIS OF ATOPIC DERMATITIS (FIG. 6-4)

1. *Dermatologic diseases.*

- *Allergic contact dermatitis.* This dermatitis results from exposure of a sensitized person to a chemical. The affected area resembles an eczematous lesion similar to the lesion in atopic dermatitis.

- *Irritant dermatitis.* Frequent hand-washing can cause an eczematous-like reaction.

- *Other eczematous lesions* such as *nummular eczema* (coin-shaped sores following skin injury or insect bites) and *dyshidrotic eczema* (itchy blisters on palms and soles that may be related to allergies or stress)

- *Stasis dermatitis* is a chronic condition that usually occurs in the lower extremities and resembles the eczema of atopic dermatitis.

- *Psoriasis* is a chronic skin condition that usually involves the elbows, knees, and gluteal folds, among other areas.

- *Acrodermatitis enteropathica* exhibits demarcated psoriasiform plaques, sometimes vesicles or bullae with usual distribution in the periorificial and acral (distal limb and head) area.

FIGURE 6-4. DIFFERENTIAL DIAGNOSIS OF ATOPIC DERMATITIS	
CATEGORY	**EXAMPLES**
Dermatologic	Allergic contact dermatitis, irritant dermatitis; nummular eczema; dyshidrotic eczema; stasis dermatitis; psoriasis; acrodermatitis enteropathica
Infectious disease	Scabies; candidiasis
Malignancies	Cutaneous T cell lymphoma (mycosis fungoides, Sezary syndrome)
Congenital Disorders	Sex-linked recessive ichthyosis caused by sulfatase deficiency; bullous congenital ichthyosiform erythroderma
Metabolic disorders	Zinc deficiency; histidine deficiency; niacin deficiency; vitamin B6 deficiency; multiple carboxylase deficiency
Immunodeficiencies	Hyper IgE syndrome; Human Immunodeficiency Virus (HIV); Wiscott- Aldrich syndrome; X-linked agammaglobulinemia; severe combined immunodeficiency syndrome; Job's syndrome; Ataxia-telangiectasia; biotinidase deficiency

2. *Infectious diseases.* Examples: *scabies, candidiasis*

3. *Malignancies.* Cutaneous T cell lymphoma (*mycosis fungoides, Sezary syndrome*)

4. *Congenital diseases. Nethertone syndrome* is an autosomal recessive disorder in newborns, characterized by red and scaly skin (*ichthyosiform erythroderma*)

5. *Metabolic disorders.* Deficiency of zinc, histidine, niacin, or vitamin B6, or *multiple carboxylase deficiency*

6. *Immunodeficiencies.* Some immunodeficiency disorders may have skin lesions that resemble atopic dermatitis. Examples are *hyper IgE syndrome; human immunodeficiency virus (HIV); Wiscott-Aldrich syndrome; X-linked agammaglobulinemia; severe combined immunodeficiency syndrome; Job's syndrome; ataxia-telangiectasia; biotinidase deficiency.*

PREVENTION AND TREATMENT OF ATOPIC DERMATITIS

The main prevention strategy is avoidance of the offending agent(s). The triggers for AD differ from one person to another, including life style differences, such as exercise, occupation, level of exposure to the offending agents, and age, among others (**Fig. 6-3**). Individuals with food allergies should eliminate the allergenic food from their diet. Those with allergic rhinitis should avoid the specific aeroallergens and undergo immunotherapy. Other measures:

1. *Hydration.* Affected patients suffer from dry skin. Heat, cold, or chemicals (e.g. soaps, detergents) may make the skin even dryer, leading to skin flareups. Therefore, hydration helps to partly reverse the dryness. Taking a bath in warm water for 20 minutes twice a day (until the fingertips wrinkle) can help moisturize the skin.

2. *Soaps.* Avoid using harsh soaps for bathing and hand washing. Also, avoid unnecessary and frequent hand washing.

3. *Moisturizers.* Use moisturizers after bathing and frequently during the day.

4. *Home and work environment.* Keep the humidity and temperature of the home and work at a comfortable range to avoid perspiration. In addition, keeping the humidity below 55% helps to keep cockroaches, dust mites, and molds away.

MEDICATIONS FOR ATOPIC DERMATITIS

1. *Corticosteroids.* The corticosteroids are grouped based on their potency (**Fig. 6-5**). Start with a mild corticosteroid such as hydrocortisone 1%. The advantage is its safety for facial use. The use of potent corticosteroids on the face is unsafe as they can cause shrinkage of skin and scarring. Mild corticosteroids are recommended for maintenance, while intermediate and high potencies are reserved for flareups.

2. *Calcineurin inhibitors.* Calcineurin is a protein phosphate that activates T cells. Calcineurin inhibitors inhibit T cell activation and belong to a class of immunosuppressants. In fact, the oral form of this medication is used for management of organ transplantation. The topical forms of calcium inhibitors, namely *tacrolimus* (prepared in ointment form) and *pimecrolimus* (prepared in cream form) are used to manage atopic dermatitis. These medications are used for two reasons. First, they are used for corticosteroid non-responsive cases. Also, they are safe for facial use in children 2 years and older.

3. *Antihistamines.* Some patients may benefit from oral antihistamines. Antihistamines are also available in topical form; however, such use is not recommended in AD, due to skin sensitization.

4. *Antibiotics.* Due to pruritus, frequent scratching, and excoriations, the eczematous skin is prone to bacterial infections, commonly *Staphylococcus aureus*. The classic infected lesion appears crusty, excoriated, and weeping, with a golden crust. These infections should be recognized and treated immediately.

5. *Phototherapy.* UV therapy is an option for resistant cases. Phototherapy targets inflammatory cells, changes

FIGURE 6-5. CLASSIFICATION OF TOPICAL CORTICOSTEROIDS		
CLASSIFICATION	**POTENCY**	**EXAMPLES - GENERIC (BRAND NAME)**
Group 1	Super potent	• clobetasol propionate 0.05% (Clobex lotion) • temovate : cream, ointment, gel • calobetasole propionate 0.05% (Ultravate) cream • fluocinonide 0.1% (Vanos cream) • betamethasone dipropionate 0.05% cream, ointment (Diprolene)
Group 2	Potent	• desoxymetasone.25% (Topicort) cream, ointment • mometasone fuorate 0.1% (Elocon) ointment
Group 3	Upper mid strength	• desoximetasone 0.05% (Topicort LP) cream • fluticasone propionate 0.005% (Cutivate) ointment
Group 4	Mid-strength	• mometasone fuorate 0.1% (Elocon) cream • fluocinolone acetonide 0.025% (Synalar) ointment
Group 5	Lower to mid-strength	• betametasone valerate 0.1% (Valisone) ointment • hydrocortisone valerate 0.2% (Westcort) ointment
Group 6	Mild	• fluocinolone acetonide 0.01% (Derma Smoothe/FS) cream • desonide 0.05% (Verdeso foam; Desonate gel)
Group 7	Least potent	• hydrocortisone 0.5%, 1% cream, spray, ointment • hydrocortisone 2.5% (Hytone) ointment, cream, lotion

cytokine production, and has an antibiotic effect in atopic dermatitis. UVB is considered an effective therapy and is available in the U.S. Combined UVA (long-wave) and UVB (short wave) or high-dose UVA1 are other alternatives. Photochemotherapy (*PUVA*) is sometimes used; it entails oral ingestion of *psoralen* (which sensitizes the skin to UV light) followed by UVA treatment. The provider should individualize the treatment based on the severity of the lesion, the therapeutic effects, and potential side effects.

A general approach to atopic dermatitis is summarized in **Figure 6-6**.

APPROACH TO ATOPIC DERMATITIS

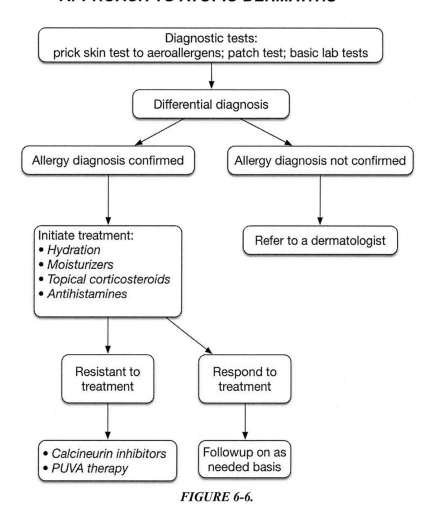

FIGURE 6-6.

Chapter 7
Allergic Contact Dermatitis

Allergic Contact Dermatitis (ACD) is an inflammation of the skin (*dermatitis*) that results from contact with an allergen.

The allergens causing ACD are contactants; i.e. they only cause an allergic reaction upon contact. Hundreds of chemicals have been identified as triggers; however, the common allergens of this type are limited.

OUTDOOR ALLERGENS

The common and important outdoor allergens are members of the plant *Anacardiceae* family. The genus *Toxicodendron* includes poison oak, poison ivy, and poison sumac. Poison ivy can grow as a shrub or grow as tall as 150 feet or trail along the ground. Poison oak is a low-growing upright shrub about 3 feet tall. Poison ivy and poison oak have a configuration of three leaves on a single stem, commonly with jagged edges. Poison sumac differs as it has a smooth-edged leaf, has about 7-10 leaves on a single reddish stem, and may grow as either a bush or tree. All three members of this family contain *urushiol*, a plant oil known to cause eczematous lesions.

OTHER ALLERGENS

Other allergens include common products found at home or work. These range from household items such as detergents; pesticides; toiletries such as soap, shampoo, perfumes, or cologne; or cosmetics such as hair dyes, foundation, lipstick, eyeliners; jewelry containing nickel; drugs (e.g. neomycin). Allergens found at work include glue, rubber products (latex gloves), paper products, and printing ink, to name a few (**Fig. 7-1**).

FIGURE 7-1. COMMON ALLERGENS CAUSING ALLERGIC CONTACT DERMATITIS	
ALLERGEN	**EXAMPLES OF PRODUCTS WITH THE ALLERGEN**
Metals:	
• Nickel sulfate	Jewelry; metal alloys; coins; scissors; keys; batteries
• Cobalt dichloride	Cements; metal tools and utensils; printing inks
• Gold sodium thiosulfate	Jewelry; gold-plate intracoronary stents; medical devices
Drugs:	
• Neomycin	Topical antibiotics; ear medications
• Bacitracin	Topical antibiotics
• Budesonide	Inhalation drugs; topical medications
• Quinoline mix	Antibacterials; antifungals
• Tixocortol-21-pivalate	Anti-inflammatories: topical medications
Cosmetics/toiletries:	
• Balsam of Peru	Perfumes and colognes; insect repellents; cleaning products
• Fragrance mix	Perfumes and colognes; scented candles; scented tobaccos
• Formaldehyde	Cosmetics: foundations; eye shadow; cleaning products; tobacco
Miscellaneous:	
• P-tert-butylphenol formaldehyde resin	Leather goods; glue; some adhesives
• Thimerosal	Fluorescent dyes; vaccines; eye drops
• Thiuram mix	Products made of natural rubber (e.g. latex gloves)

CLINICAL PRESENTATION OF ALLERGIC CONTACT DERMATITIS

In acute allergic contact dermatitis, there are pruritus, erythema, and vesiculation. Thickening of the skin occurs in chronic contact dermatitis (**Plate 5-2**).

Commonly, a teenage boy presents with erythema and rash on the upper and lower extremities on Monday. The history reveals that he was hiking on the weekend, a common presentation of ACD due to poison ivy.

Another common doctor visit is when a female patient presents on Monday with facial irritation and erythema. The history reveals that she had used a makeup sample in the shopping mall on the weekend.

PATHOPHYSIOLOGY OF ACD

Affected individuals have a history of prior exposure to the allergen, which "sensitizes" the individual. Subsequent exposure to the same allergen elicits the allergic symptoms. Allergic contact dermatitis is considered a Gell-Coombs Type IV type allergy. This type of allergy is also known as *cell-mediated* or *delayed type*. First, effector lymphocytes, CD4+ T helper cells and CD8+ T cells, are activated by antigen-presenting cells (APC, which could be macrophages, B lymphocytes or a number of other kinds of cells). As a result of this activation, the T cells release cytokines such as interferon-gamma, which activate macrophages, leading to tissue inflammation and injury (**Fig. 2-11**).

DIFFERENTIAL DIAGNOSIS OF ACD

- *Irritant contact dermatitis (ICD)* results from an exposure to irritants such as soaps or detergents. Frequent hand washing or wearing gloves for a long period of time are two examples of such triggers. An irritation aggravates the area of contact, resulting in skin cracking, oozing and possible secondary infection. In the mild form of ICD, the skin appears erythematous and dry, with fissuring. Individuals with irritant contact dermatitis are prone to allergic contact dermatitis, because the allergens can easily penetrate the skin and start the cascade of sensitization and allergic reaction.

- *Atopic dermatitis* is the lesion in atopic individuals. It presents as an eczematous (erythematous, scaly, and vesicular) rash (see **Chapter 6**).

- *Fungal infections* include *Tinea pedis* (a cause of fungal infection in the feet) and *Tinea corporis* (a cause of fungal infection on the body). *Tinea pedis* starts in web spaces of the toes and presents as peeling with maceration associated with pruritus. *Tinea corporis*, also known as "*ring worm*," is a superficial fungal infection that presents as a round, ringed lesion, erythematous with central clearing and scaly border.

- *Mycosis fungoides*, also known as *cutaneous T-cell lymphoma*, originates from the skin. It has a *premycotic phase* (scaly, red rash on body areas not generally exposed to sun), a *patch phase* (a thin, red, eczematous rash), a *plaque phase* (small, raised bumps or hardened, often reddened, areas on the skin, followed by a *tumor phase*, which may ulcerate and become infected.

DIAGNOSIS OF ALLERGIC CONTACT DERMATITIS

History

Due to delayed presentation of this type of allergy, the examiner should obtain a history of contact with potential allergens in the previous 2–7 days. The following are common questions based on anatomical body parts:

1. *Head (scalp irritation, rash)*: Have you used a new hair dye, a new shampoo, a new hair conditioner?

Comment: *Paraben mix*, a preservative used in many hair colors, is a cause of contact dermatitis.

2. *Eyes/Eyelids:* Are you using goggles? Are you using an ophthalmic medication (eye drops, cream, or ointment)? Are you using an eye shadow, eyeliner or any eye mascara?

Comment: Goggles may contain *thiuram mix* (used in processing latex), a cause of contact dermatitis. Some eye drop medications use an antiseptic, *thimerosal*, as a preservative. *Quaternium-15* and *formaldehyde* are used in some eye shadows, eyeliners and eye pencils.

3. *Ears:* Are you using any aural medication? *Neomycin* and *bacitracin* are two examples of potentially allergic medications.

4. Are you using new earrings? A very common culprit is nickel-containing jewelry. Gold earrings are another example.

5. Are you using a new hearing aid? Hearing aids containing acrylic material can cause ACD.

6. *Nose*: Are you wearing any piercing jewelry? Neomycin and bacitracin used externally can cause allergic reactions, as can *budesonide* nasal spray (for asthma).

7. Are you using any lotion, sunscreen, foundation, or powder on the nose?

8. *Oropharynx:* Have you been using anything on the lips such as lipstick or lotion? *Paraben mix* is an example of a potentially allergenic preservative used in lipsticks.

9. Have you worn pierced jewelry on your lips or tongue?

10. Do you use a denture? Glue used for the denture may be allergenic.

11. *Face:* Do you use any facial cosmetics, like foundations, powder, lotions, perfumes, or sunscreen?

12. *Waist:* Sometimes patients present with dermatitis around the waist. Do your underpants have elastic rubber material? Elastics used in underpants may contain latex, which can cause ACD.

13. *Hands:* Are you wearing any new jewelry or using a new cream or lotion?

14. Do you use latex gloves? Latex gloves contain *thiuram mix* and *mercapto mix*, potential allergens.

15. *Skin:* Have you been using a new laundry detergent? Are you using a new body wash, soap, or sunscreen? Allergens may come in contact with any area of the skin. The severity and presentation of reactions depend on the product used, the area of exposure and duration of the contact. For example, using sunscreen before swimming covers a larger body surface area than an eyeliner. Some skin areas are more sensitive than others, e.g. the eyelids, which have thinner skin compared to the scalp or palms.

Every time we use a new skin product, we risk sensitization and future expression of an allergic contact dermatitis.

Diagnostic Testing for Allergic Contact Dermatitis

ACD is a delayed reaction. The initial reaction manifests approximately 48 hours after the first contact and may become more pronounced 2-4 days later. The idea of testing is to expose the allergen to the skin and observe the delayed reaction. This test, known as the *patch test*

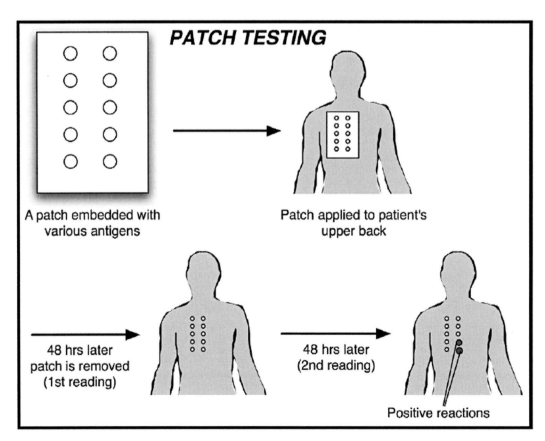

PATCH TESTING

A patch embedded with various antigens

Patch applied to patient's upper back

48 hrs later patch is removed (1st reading)

48 hrs later (2nd reading)

Positive reactions

FIGURE 7-2. (From Mahmoudi, M. Immunology Made Ridiculously Simple, Medmaster)

is commercially available for over 30 common allergens. The steps in performing the test are (**Fig. 7-2**):

- Cleanse the upper back with alcohol.
- Apply the allergen-embedded self-adhesive patch to the area.
- Secure the patch to prevent it from coming off due to sweating or movement.
- Mark the area to identify the orientation of the patches.
- Instruct the patient to avoid wetting the area.
- The first visit for preliminary observation of the reaction is 48 hours post-application.
- On the first visit, the patch is removed, and irritation, inflammation, or blister formation is recorded.
- The second observation is 1-2 days after the first visit (72-96 hours after the initial application).
- On the second visit, the area of the patch contact is observed and the reactions are recorded. A positive reaction ranges from a mild erythema and papules to vesicles, blisters, or bullae.

PREVENTION/TREATMENT OF ALLERGIC CONTACT DERMATITIS

- Identification and avoidance of the allergen is the best method of prevention. This can be accomplished with a thorough history and patch testing.
- Liberal use of moisturizers
- Burow's solution (aluminum acetate solution)
- Oatmeal baths provide relief.
- Wet dressing covering the affected areas
- Topical corticosteroids, mild potency corticosteroids for the face and medium-to-high potency for other body parts (**Fig. 6-5**)
- In steroid non-responsive cases, or when mild corticosteroids are not effective on the face, topical calcineurin inhibitors may be a reasonable alternative.
- Oral steroids, phototherapy with PUVA or narrowband UVB is reserved for chronic conditions unresponsive to initial therapy.

Chapter 8

Asthma

Asthma is a chronic inflammatory disease of the airways. It is characterized by respiratory symptoms (shortness of breath, wheezing or cough), airway inflammation, airway obstruction, and hyperresponsiveness (an exaggerated bronchoconstriction caused by a wide variety of stimuli). In 2009, approximately 25 million people had asthma in the United States. This is a tremendous increase from about 20 million in 2001. In 2012, 8% of the adult population (18 years and over) and 9.3% of children had asthma. The number of asthmatics worldwide is estimated at 300 million, of whom 250,000 deaths are reported every year.

Asthmatics present with one or more symptoms of shortness of breath, chest tightness, wheezing, or cough, which may be the only presenting symptom (**Fig. 8-1**). Asthma presenting with cough as the only airway symptom is known as *cough variant asthma*.

FIGURE 8-1. CLINICAL PRESENTATION OF ASTHMA	
Subjective Factors	Shortness of breath, wheezing, cough
Objective factors	Wheezing, reduced ventilation
Airway abnormalities	Obstruction (partial or complete); increased hyperresponsiveness to various stimuli (e.g. pollens, pet dander, smoke)

TYPES OF ASTHMA

There are several types of asthma. Each type starts at a different age and is triggered by specific agents (**Fig. 8-2**):

- *Allergic Asthma* is the most common type of asthma. It starts in childhood and may resolve in a few years or recur later in life (in the 20's) and continue for life. The patients become symptomatic after exposure to aeroallergens. Affected individuals have abnormal lung function tests and require medical management. A subset of patients presents with asthma symptoms but has normal lung function tests. The affected individuals become symptomatic after brief exposure to aeroallergens (*respiratory allergy*). The treatment of allergic asthma includes allergy immunotherapy, targeting specific allergens, and customized medication management (see therapy section in this chapter and immunotherapy **Chapter 11**).

FIGURE 8-2. TYPES OF ASTHMA, AGE OF ONSET, AND TRIGGERS		
TYPES OF ASTHMA	AGE OF ONSET	TRIGGERS
Allergic asthma	Usually childhood	Aeroallergens: e.g. pollens, dust mites, animal dander, mold spores
Adult onset asthma	Adulthood	Unknown, various stimuli
Occupational asthma	Adulthood	Various triggers in work environment
Exercise-induced asthma	Any age	Exercise, strenuous activities (e.g. climbing stairs)
Aspirin-induced asthma	Any age	Aspirin and other non-steroid anti-inflammatory drugs (NSAIDs)
Cough variant asthma	Any age	Unknown
Mixed asthma (asthma+ COPD)	Late adulthood	Unknown -- depends on type of asthma

- *Adult Onset Asthma* starts in adulthood. Its etiology is unknown. The workup includes lung function tests and allergy skin testing, but the results of allergy testing are usually negative.

- *Occupational Asthma* comprises approximately 10% of all asthma; it is characterized by airway hyperresponsiveness and airway obstruction due to agent(s) specifically related to the work environment. Many agents can cause occupational asthma; they are divided into high and low molecular weight agents, immunologic agents, and non-immunologic agents, such as irritant gases and some chemicals.

The high molecular weight agents include animal or plant proteins, enzymes, and natural rubber latex. These agents are larger than 1000 KD (kilodalton). The low molecular weight agents include isocyanates, such as naphthalene, some drugs, wood dust, amines, formaldehyde and ethylene oxide (**Fig. 8-3**).

FIGURE 8-3. CAUSATIVE AGENTS OF OCCUPATIONAL ASTHMA				
AGENTS	**TYPE**	**EXAMPLES (AGENTS)**	**EXAMPLES (PROFESSIONS)**
High Molecular Weight	Animal proteins	Animal dander; insect scales; fish; other seafood	Veterinarian; laboratory personnel; researchers; farmers; poultry processors
	Plant proteins	Wheat; grains; dusts; castor beans; coffee beans; guar gum; latex	Bakers; farmers; greenhouse workers
	Enzymes	From bacillus subtilis; baking enzymes	Health care providers; toy manufacturers; washing powder industry; bakers
Low Molecular Weight	Drugs	Beta lactate agents; opiates; piperazine	Pharmaceutical personnel; health professionals
	Isocyanates	Naphthalene diisocyanate; hexamethylene diisocyanate	Roofers; insulators
	Metals	Nickle sulfate; platinum salts	Metal workers
	Wood dust	Red cedar	Carpenters; sawmill workers; forestry workers
Irritants	Gases, fumes	Chlorine; anhydrous ammonia	Laboratory personnel

Sometimes, workers are exposed to non-immunologic agents (irritants). Symptoms from this type of exposure are referred to as *Reactive Airway Dysfunction Syndrome (RADS)*. This type of reaction results from a single exposure to a high dose of irritant, such as chlorine.

- In *Exercise-induced Asthma (EIA)*, affected individuals become symptomatic after exercise or strenuous activity. This condition is also called *exercise-induced bronchospasm* or *exercise-induced airway narrowing*. EIA is common; its prevalence in asthmatics has been reported to be as high as 90%. Affected individuals present with typical asthma symptoms, such as shortness of breath, chest tightness, wheezing, and cough. However, the examiner should also pay attention to atypical symptoms such as chest pain, fatigue and stomach aches. EIA can present alone or can manifest in other type of asthma. For example, an individual with allergic asthma may also experience asthma symptoms with exercise.

- In *Aspirin-induced Asthma (AIA)*, ingestion of aspirin or other non-steroidal anti-inflammatory drugs (NSAIDs) results in respiratory symptoms. AIA is a clinical syndrome that is commonly associated with rhinosinusitis, nasal polyposis, aspirin sensitivity, and asthma. The reaction starts within 3 hours of ingestion.

- *Mixed Asthma.* Asthmatics sometimes present with a mixed picture of asthma and COPD (Chronic Obstructive Pulmonary Disease). Such individuals usually become asthmatic first. With progression of the asthma, especially if not treated, the airways lose their elasticity, become floppy and collapsible, and develop a COPD-like picture. To follow the trend of the asthmas's progression, one can review and compare a series of lung function tests (e.g. *spirometry*). Lung function tests that show reversibility of the airway symptoms after use of a bronchodilator gradually change to demonstrate less or no reversibility. In both asthma and COPD the patient has difficulty blowing air out (they are both *obstructive airway diseases*). An asthma attack, though, is reversible with the proper treatment.

PATHOGENESIS OF ASTHMA

Some asthma triggers have been identified and may have different mechanisms. *Aeroallergens* are one of the most studied of these triggers. An allergen can cause differentiation of the naïve T helper cells to the subset of T helper cells known as Th2. Th2 cells produce interleukin 4 (IL-4), interleukin 5 (IL-5), and interleukin 13 (IL-13). IL-4 stimulates B cells, which leads to production of IgE; IL-5 activates eosinophils; IL-13 acts similarly to IL-4. IgE binds to the high affinity receptor (FceRI) on the surface of mast cells. After repeated exposure to the same aeroallergen, and the influence of Th2 and B cells, the mast cells degranulate (**Fig. 2-6**). Various chemical mediators are released from mast cells (**Fig. 2-5**). The actions of these mediators include:

- Histamine and leukotrienes (C4, D4, and E4) cause bronchospasm.

- Prostaglandin D2 (PGD2) increases vascular permeability and stimulates neutrophil chemotaxis (attracts neutrophils).

- Interleukin 5 (IL5) stimulates eosinophil production, activation, growth, and differentiation.

The interplay of these mediators from mast cells and eosinophils results in bronchospasm and airway inflammation.

Respiratory infection also plays a role in the pathogenesis of asthma. Infection of humans with viruses such as Respiratory Syncytial Virus (RSV), parainfluenza virus, and rhinoviruses can cause respiratory symptoms. In the mild form of the illness, affected individual may suffer from an acute upper respiratory infection. However, if the virus penetrates to the lower airway, it could result in wheezing with bronchitis or pneumonia. Obstruction of the lower airway can eventually lead to asthma.

DIAGNOSIS OF ASTHMA

History

The following are selected questions that can be used to diagnose the affected patient. These questions may be discussed face-to-face or written out before the doctor visit.

1. How do you describe your breathing? Are you short of breath? Do you have chest tightness? Do you cough? How about wheezing?
2. How often do you experience your symptoms? Are they daily?
3. Do your respiratory symptoms waken you at night? If so, how often? How many nights are you awakened per week?
4. Have you identified the triggers of your respiratory symptoms? If not, how about the following:

   a. Do your symptoms start outdoors (after exposure to pollens)?
   b. Do your symptoms start indoors (after exposure to pets, dusts, molds)?
   c. Do you have pets? Specifically, do you have a cat or a bird?
   d. Do your symptoms start after exercise or strenuous activities?
   e. Does cold weather bring on your symptoms?

   The following questions are tailored for younger children and can be addressed to a parent:

5. Does your child become short of breath after crying or laughing?
6. Is your child active in physical education classes?
7. Can your child keep up with the pace of peers in physical education classes?

Physical Examination

General observation of the patient helps us to suspect respiratory pathology. For example, does the patient appear to be short of breath while walking to the exam room? Does the patient have audible wheezing? On auscultation of the lungs, the examiner should pay attention to air ventilation, abnormal audible sounds, specifically wheezing (musical sounds), but also other respiratory sounds, such as rhonchi (coarse sounds) or rales (fine crackling sounds).

Diagnostic Tests For Asthma

Chest X-ray. Unless you suspect pneumonia or heart failure, chest x-ray is not essential for diagnosis. Regardless, a chest x-ray usually shows hyperinflation.

Spirometry. The patient's lung function is measured by using a simple portable *spirometer* machine. Measuring lung function with a spirometer is a patient-dependent task. Since the results of spirometry represent the status of the patient's lung function, every effort should be made to ensure that the result is not altered by the technical operation of the device. The test is usually done three times, and the best measurement is automatically selected. Before the test, patient identification information is obtained and recorded in the machine, including name, age, race, height, weight, and smoking history. This collected information (especially race, age, and height) is important because it should be compared with normal values of the like group already stored in the spirometry memory. For example, the lung function of a 15-year-old white male should be compared with predicted normal values of other 15-year-old white males.

During a spirometry test, ask the patient to:

1. Take a deep breath and fill lungs with air.
2. Place the mouth around the mouthpiece to seal it. Some recommend placing the mouthpiece between the teeth and using a nose clip to keep the nostrils closed.
3. Blow as *hard and as fast* as possible until feeling that there is no more air to blow out.

Note: Some spirometry machines have a beeping sound that directs the patient to blow more air. Then the patient should be instructed to follow the beeping sound.

4. While the mouth is still on the mouthpiece, inhale as hard as possible.
5. Repeat steps 1-4 three times.
6. The best test measurement is selected by the machine and printed. The generated graph is interpreted by the physician.

Interpretation of the Spirometry Result

First we need to be familiar with lung volume and lung capacity. The following is basic terminology (**Fig. 8-4**):

- *Tidal Volume (VT)*. This is the volume of air in a normal inhalation/exhalation respiratory cycle.
- *Inspiratory Reserve Volume (IRV)*. This is the maximum volume of air inhaled after a normal inhalation.
- *Expiratory Reserve Volume (ERV)* is the forced exhaled volume of air after a normal exhalation.
- *Residual Volume (RV)* is the volume of air left in the lung after a deep exhalation.
- *Inspiratory Capacity (IC)* is the maximum volume of air inhaled after a normal exhalation.
- *Functional Residual Capacity (FRC)* is the volume of air remaining after a normal exhalation.
- *Vital Capacity (VC)* is the maximum volume of air that can be exhaled after a maximum inhalation. It is the sum of Tidal Volume (VT), Inspiratory Reserve Volume (IRV) and Expiratory Reserve Volume (ERV). VC = VT + IRV + ERV

- *Total Lung Capacity (TLC)* is the maximum volume of air in the lungs, which is the sum of Inspiratory Reserve Volume (IRV), Tidal Volume (VT), Expiratory Reserve Volume (ERV), and Residual Volume (RV).

The following are commonly measured or calculated parameters that help interpret the result:

A. *Peak Expiratory Flow Rate (PEF)*. This is the maximum speed of forced expiration after a deep breath.

B. *Forced vital capacity (FVC)*. This is the amount of air that is exhaled after a deep inhalation.

C. *Forced expiratory volume in one second (FEV1)*. This is the amount of air that is exhaled forcefully in the first second.

D. *The ratio of FEV1/FVC.*

E. *FEF 25-75% (Forced expiratory flow volume)* is the area of curve that represents 25% exhalation of FVC to 75% exhalation of FVC. This measurement represents the function of the small airways.

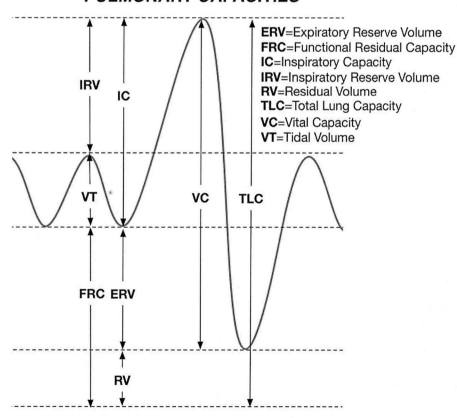

PULMONARY CAPACITIES

ERV=Expiratory Reserve Volume
FRC=Functional Residual Capacity
IC=Inspiratory Capacity
IRV=Inspiratory Reserve Volume
RV=Residual Volume
TLC=Total Lung Capacity
VC=Vital Capacity
VT=Tidal Volume

FIGURE 8-4. Spirometry terminology.

PEF gives an overall picture of respiratory function. Those with airway obstruction are unable to reach the normal values.

FVC. A normal airway is expected to have an FVC of at least 80% of predicted values. This number is reduced in individuals with asthma and chronic obstructive pulmonary disease (COPD). When interpreting the value of FVC, the measurement of FEV1 should also be considered and compared.

FEV1/FVC (also known as FEV1%). This ratio is used as a marker of obstruction. A normal lung is expected to have a ratio of at least 80%. However, one has to be careful interpreting this ratio. For example, the lung function may be abnormal and still show a ratio of 100%, with an FEV1of 70 and FVC of 70. Although each value is reduced, the ratio is still 100%. An FEV1/FVC ratio of less than 70% indicates airway obstruction.

FEF 25-75%. As mentioned, this measurement represents the respiratory flow status of the smaller airways. Reduced numbers just show an abnormal lung function.

In order to diagnose asthma by spirometry, the spirometry should be repeated 15-30 minutes after using a short-acting bronchodilator such as an albuterol inhaler. The measured numbers, post-bronchodilator, should be compared with pre-bronchodilator measurement. Asthma is diagnosed when FEV1 increases by at least 12% and 200 ml post-bronchodilator. The spirometry test results are presented by two diagrams: a flow volume loop that is graphed as flow (liters/second) versus volume in liters (**Fig. 8-5**) and a volume/time curve in which volume in liters is graphed versus time in seconds (**Fig. 8-6**).

Restrictive lung diseases are disorders in which the lungs resist expansion; there is difficulty getting air into the lungs. Causes include intrinsic lung disease (e.g. asbestosis, sarcoidosis), chest wall resistance (e.g. scoliosis), and neuromuscular disease (e.g. muscular dystrophy). There are reduced FVC and FEV1 in restrictive lung disease, but *normal or elevated* FEV1/FVC, since, while FEV1 is decreased, total lung capacity is also significantly decreased. In asthma and obstructive lung disease, though, total lung capacity is not decreased, so FEV1/FVC is *decreased.*

Examples of a normal spirogram, an asthmatic spirogram, and a restriction pattern are illustrated in **Figure 8-7**.

Exhaled Nitric Oxide (NO). Nitric Oxide (NO) gas is not only found in pollutants from motor vehicle exhausts and cigarette smoke, but is also produced by human lungs. NO functions as a vasodilator, bronchodilator, neurotransmitter, and inflammatory mediator. It has been shown that asthmatic lungs produce higher levels of NO compared to normal lungs. Consideration of this fact has led to the design of a device for measuring exhaled NO in those with suspected asthma. The American Thoracic Society has recommended the measurement of exhaled NO in the diagnosis of eosinophilic airway inflammation, for determining the likelihood of steroid responsiveness in individuals with chronic respiratory symptoms possibly due to airway inflammation, and also to support the diagnosis of asthma in which objective evidence is needed.

The following is the 2011 recommendation of the interpretation of Exhaled Nitric Oxide Level (FeNO) of the American Thoracic Society Clinical Practice Guideline (**Fig. 8-8**):

FENO (fractional nitric oxide in exhaled breath) < 25 ppb (part per billion) in adults (< 20 ppb for children under 12 years old) suggests that both eosinophilic inflammation and responsiveness to corticosteroids are less likely.

FENO > 50 ppb in adults or > 35 ppb in children suggests the likelihood of eosinophilic inflammation and responsiveness to corticosteroids.

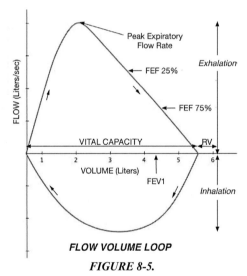

FLOW VOLUME LOOP

FIGURE 8-5.

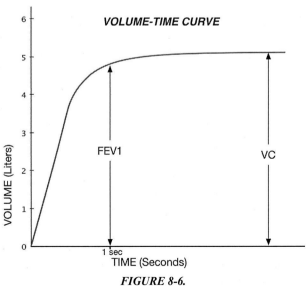

FIGURE 8-6.

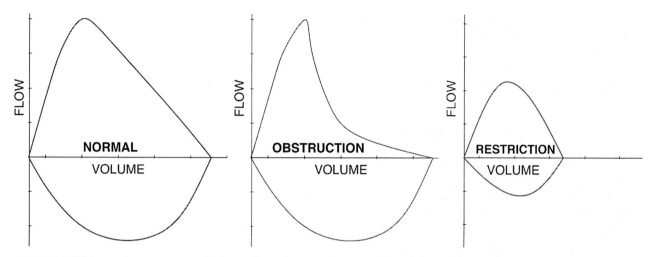

FIGURE 8-7. Three spirograms: normal, obstructive pulmonary disease, and restrictive pulmonary disease.

FENO between 25-50 ppb in adults and 25-35 ppb in children should be interpreted cautiously, with reference to the clinical context.

Although some allergists use the FENO measurement in asthmatics, this measurement is not widely used because:

FIGURE 8-8. RECOMMENDED INTERPRETATION OF MEASURED FE_{NO}		
FE_{NO} = fractional nitric oxide in exhaled breath; ppb = part per billion Adopted from American Thoracic Society Clinical Practice Guideline (2011)		
FE_{NO} (PPB) RANGE FOR ADULT	FE_{NO} (PPB) RANGE FOR CHILDREN UNDER 12 YEARS OLD	LIKELIHOOD OF EOSINOPHILIC INFLAMMATION/ CORTICOSTEROID RESPONSIVENESS
< 25	< 20	Less likely
>50	>35	Likely
Between 25-50	Between 20-35	Should be interpreted cautiously with reference to the clinical circumstances.

1. Spirometry is still the single best method for measuring lung function; it is widely available and affordable, and is a sufficient diagnostic test for asthma when done pre and post use of a bronchodilator.

2. The FENO analyzers are considered a supplementary tool for diagnosis of asthma and cannot substitute for spirometry measurement.

3. The FENO analyzer is an expensive device especially for providers who do not see enough patients, and it is not cost-effective.

4. The FENO test is not widely accepted by the insurance companies.

5. There is low reimbursement from insurance companies.

PREVENTION AND TREATMENT OF ASTHMA

Prevention of Asthma

- Take your medications regularly.
- Avoid cold weather, wear warm clothes, and especially cover your face to avoid direct exposure to cold.
- Avoid pollutants and cigarette smoke.
- Avoid aspirin and other non-steroid anti-inflammatory drugs (NSAIDs) if you have aspirin-induced asthma; read over-the-counter medication labels.
- If you have exercise-induced asthma, use your short-acting bronchodilator (e.g. albuterol inhaler) 15 to 30 minutes before exercise.
- If you have allergic asthma, avoid outdoor activity on high pollen days.
- When you have an asthma flareup, increase the dose of your corticosteroid inhaler or add another medication based on your "asthma action plan" discussed below.

Treatment of Asthma

Ashma medications are delivered in several forms: oral (tablets), inhalers such as metered dose inhalers (MDI), dry powder inhalers (DPI), nebulizers, and injectable.

Metered dose inhalers (MDI) use a chemical propellant to push the medication out of the inhaler. In the past,

MDIs contained *chlorofluorocarbon (CFC)*, but these were phased out and replaced by *hydrofluoroalkane inhalers (HFA)*, because the CFC inhalers harmed the environment by reducing the protective ozone layer. Based on an international agreement, the *Montreal Protocol on Substances That Deplete the Ozone Layer*, the HFA MDIs replaced the CFC MDIs.

Dry powder inhalers (DPI) do not contain propellant. The medication is in the form of dry powder. Since there is no propellant in the device, the DPI is "breath-activated" to release the drug from the device.

Diskus, a dry powder device, features a built-in counter that shows the number inhalations remaining after each use.

Nebulizers deliver the medication in the form of a mist, via a mask or mouthpiece.

There are two classes of medication for asthma management, *Rescuers* and *Controllers*.

Rescuers are medications that are used for immediate relief of asthma symptoms; these are short-acting bronchodilators (e.g. an albuterol inhaler). *Albuterol* and *levalbuterol* are beta-2 agonists which bind to beta-2 receptors in the lung and causes bronchodilation. The anticholinergic *ipratropium bromide* in inhaler form is used as a single drug or in combination with albuterol (**Fig. 8-9**).

Controllers are for long-term management of asthma symptoms and are often continued for life. These are mainly *corticosteroid inhalers*, anti-inflammatory topical medications that are either used alone or in combination with long-acting bronchodilators (**Fig. 8-10**).

One class of controllers is *leukotriene inhibitors*. Leukotrienes are lipid inflammatory mediators synthesized in and released from mast cells and basophils, among other sources. They can induce bronchospasm; increased vascular permeability; and constriction of arterial, arteriolar and intestinal smooth muscle. Therefore, leukotriene inhibitors, which are non-inhaled controller medications, have anti-inflammatory and bronchodilatory effect. There are two subclasses of these inhibitors: *leukotriene receptor antagonists* and *5-lipoxygenase inhibitors* (**Fig. 8-11**), which are used in the treatment of asthma as well as prevention for exercise-induced bronchospasm. Leukotrienes are usually used in combination with a corticosteroid inhaler; however, leukotriene receptor antagonists can also be used alone in step 2 management of asthma for children 5 to 11 years old and adults 12 years and older (**Figs. 8-12** and **8-13**).

Omalizumab is an anti-IgE antibody that is indicated for moderate to severe persistent asthma in patients 12 years of age and older. Omalizumab is a monoclonal antibody that binds to the FcεRI (high affinity receptor) binding site on the free IgE molecules and forms an IgE-anti-IgE complex. As a result of this binding, less free IgE

FIGURE 8-9. BRONCHODILATORS				
DRUG	**MECHANISM**	**DELIVERY SYSTEM**	**INDICATION**	**DOSE**
Albuterol	Beta-2 agonist Nebulizer 0.63 mg/3ml; 1.25 mg/3 ml; 2.5 mg/3ml 0.5%	Metered dose inhaler	Used prophylactically to prevent exercise–induced asthma; immediate relief of bronchospasm	4 years or older: • 1-2 inhalations 15-30 minutes before exercise • 1-2 inhalations every 4-6 hours as needed
		Bronchospasm	2 years or older: • I vial by nebulizer 3-4 times/day over 5-15 minutes • Not recommended for adults	
		Bronchospasm	3-4 times/day (adult only)	
Levalbuterol	Beta-2 agonist (single isomer albuterol) Nebulizer 0.31 mg/ 3ml; 0.63 mg/3ml; 1.25 mg/ 3ml	Metered dose inhaler	Bronchospasm	4 years or older: • 2 inhalation every 4-6 hours
		Bronchospasm	6-11 years old: 0.31 mg 3 times a day Adult: 0.63 mg 3 times a day, 6-8 hour intervals	
Ipatropium bromide	Anticholinergic	Metered dose inhaler	Bronchospasm (use as an alternative bronchodilator if beta-2 agonist not tolerated)	2 inhalations 4 times a day as needed

FIGURE 8-10. CORTICOSTEROID INHALERS MDI = METERED DOSE INHALER				
MEDICATION	**ACTIVE INGRE-DIENT**	**METHOD OF DELIVERY**	**DOSE (CHILDREN 4-11 YR)**	**DOSE (12 YRS & OLDER)**
Fluticasone propionate: MDI inhaler: 44 mcg, 110 mcg, 220 mcg Diskus inhaler; 50 mcg, 110 mcg, 250 mcg)	Corticosteroid	MDI Diskus inhaler	MDI: 2 inhalations of 44 mcg bid (aerosol) Diskus: 1 inhalation of 50 mcg bid	MDI: 2 inhalations of 44 mcg bid Diskus: 1 inhalation of 100 mcg bid
Beclomethasone dipropionate (40, 80 mcg)/inhalation)	Corticosteroid	MDI	5 -11 years: 1 inhalation of 40 mcg bid	1-2 inhalations of 40 mcg bid
Budesonide (90, 180 mcg/inhalation)	Corticosteroid	Dry powder	6 yrs or older: 1 inhalation of 180 mcg bid	18 yrs or older: 1 or 2 inhalations of 180 mcg bid
Flunisolide	Corticosteroid	MDI	6-15 yrs: 2 inhalations bid	2 inhalations bid
Mometasone (110 , 220 mcg/inhalation)	Corticosteroid	MDI	110 mcg, 1 inhalation in pm	220 mcg, 1 inhalation in pm
Ciclesonide (80, 160 mcg/inhalation)	Corticosteroid	MDI	Not recommended	1 inhalation of 80 mcg bid
Fluticasone + salmeterol: MDI: (45 mcg/21 mcg; 115 mcg /21 mcg; 230 mcg /21 mcg) Diskus: (100mcg/50 mcg: 250mcg /50 mcg; 500 mcg /50 mcg)	Corticosteroid + long-acting beta-2 agonist	MDI Diskus	MDI: 1 inhalation of 100/50 bid Diskus not recommended	HFA: 2 inhalations of 45/21, 115/21, or 230/21 bid Diskus: 1 inhalation of 100/50 or 250/50 bid
Mometasone furoate + formoterol fumarate: (110 mcg/5 mcg; 200 mcg/ 5 mcg)	Corticosteroid + long acting beta-2-agonist	MDI	Not recommended	2 inhalations bid
Budesonide + formoterol fumarate: (80mcg/4.5mcg; 160 mcg/4.5 mcg)	Corticosteroid + long-acting beta-2 agonist	Pressurized MDI	Not recommended	2 inhalations of 80/4.5 or 160/4.5 bid

becomes available for binding to the FcεRI binding sites of the mast cells. The anti-IgE antibody is commercially available in an injectable form. The medication dosage is calculated based on total serum IgE and body weight, and is administered every 2-4 weeks.

Theophylline is a unique medication. It is a xanthine derivative with two distinct activities: It acts as a bronchodilator and prophylactically suppresses the response of the airways to stimuli. However, due to its toxicity and interaction with many drugs, it has limited usage in modern asthma treatment.

Treatment of asthma is based on frequency of symptoms, frequency of using a short-acting bronchodilator, interference of symptoms with daily activity, and lung function. Using this information, the Expert Panel Report 3 of the National Asthma Education and Prevention Program of the National Heart, Lung, and Blood Institute (2007) has classified asthma into *intermittent, mild persistent, moderate persistent* and *severe persistent* forms (**Fig. 8-14**). Once the diagnosis is established, the panel recommends a stepwise approach for treatment (**Figs. 8-12 and 8-13**).

While on therapy, the patient should be followed for examination and spirometry to assess the possibility of a step-down regimen. In other words, when the patient's condition improves, the patient may need less medication

			FIGURE 8-11. NON-INHALER ASTHMA CONTROLLER MEDICATIONS		
MEDICATION	**FORMS**	**MECHANISM**	**DOSE**	**COMMENT**
Montelukast	Granules, 5 and 10 mg tablets	Leukotriene receptor antagonist	• 12-23 months: 4 mg chew tablet or granule packet in the evening • 2-5 yrs: 4 mg chew tablet or granule in the evening • 6-14 yrs: 5 mg tablet in evening • 15 yrs and older: 10 mg tablet once in evening	For exercise-induced bronchospasm, take at least 2 hrs before exercise (patient 6 years of age or older)
Zafirlukast	10 and 20 mg tablets	Leukotriene receptor antagonist	• Younger than 5 yrs: not recommended • 5-11 yrs: 10 mg bid • Adult: 20 mg bid	Take 1hr before or 2 hr after meal. Contraindicated in active liver disease and persistent ALT elevations.
Zileuton	600 mg tablet	5-Lipoxygenase inhibitor	• Children: not recommended • Adult:1 tab qid	Take 4 times/day with meals and at bedtime
Omalizumab	Injectable	Anti-IgE inhibitor	• Children: Not recommended • 12 yrs and older: dosage based on total IgE and body weight	
Theophylline (Extended release)	Oral	Bronchodilator	Consult package insert. Dose based on age and weight	Check serum level for dose adjustments
Mepolizumab	Injectable (subcutaneous)	Interleukin-5 antagonist; a monoclonal antibody	• Children under 12 yrs: not recommended • 12 yrs and older 100 mg subcutaneously every 4 weeks injection	Medication is for Rx of ages 12 yrs & older with severe asthma with eosinophilic phenotype

FIGURE 8-12. *STEPWISE APPROACH TO ASTHMA MANAGEMENT AGES 5-11 YEARS*

ICS= inhaled corticosteroid; LABA= inhaled long-acting beta-2 agonist; LTRA= leukotriene receptor antagonist; SABA= short-acting beta-2 agonist. Based on the Expert Panel report 3 of the National Heart, Lung, and Blood Institute (2007).

STEPS	SABA	ICS	LABA	OMALI-ZUMAB	LTRA	THEOPHYLLINE	ORAL STEROID	COMMENT
1	+							As needed
2		Low dose						Or use cromolyn , LTRA, nedocromil or theophylline
3		Low dose	+		+	+		Add either LABA, LTRA, or theophylline to low dose ICS Or use medium dose ICS only
4		Medium dose	+					Alternative: medium dose ICS + LTRA or theophylline
5		High dose	+					Alternative: high dose ICS + LTRA or high dose ICS + theophylline
6		High dose	+				+	Alternative: high dose ICS + LTRA or theophylline + oral corticosteroids

and therefore may climb down the management steps as described in **Figures 8-12** and **8-13**. In addition, immunotherapy is considered for those with allergic asthma.

New Medications

More recently, another class of medication was approved by the Food and Drug Administration. Interleukin-5 (IL-5) is involved in eosinophil maturation and survival. In view of the importance of eosinophils in asthma, a monoclonal antibody against IL-5 has been used in severe asthmatics with the eosinophilic phenotype. It is injectable and administered every 4 weeks.

FIGURE 8-13. STEPWISE APPROACH TO ASTHMA MANAGEMENT AGE 12 AND OLDER

ICS= inhaled corticosteroid; LABA= inhaled long-acting beta-2 agonist; LTRA= leukotriene receptor antagonist; SABA= short-acting beta-2 agonist. Based on the Expert Panel report 3 of the National Heart, Lung, and Blood Institute (2007).

STEPS	SABA	ICS	LABA	OMALIZUMAB	ORAL STEROID	COMMENT
1	+					As needed
2		Low dose				Alternative: cromolyn , LTRA, nedocromil or theophyline
3		Low dose	+			Or medium dose ICS Alternative: Low dose ICS + either LTRA, theophylline or zileuton
4		Medium dose	+			Alternative: medium dose ICS + either LTRA, theophylline or zileuton
5		High dose	+	+ (consideration for patients with allergies)	+	
6		High dose	+	+ (consideration for patients with allergies)	+	

FIGURE 8-14. CLASSIFICATION OF ASTHMA SEVERITY AGE 12 AND OLDER

FEV1 = forced expiratory volume in 1 second; FVC = Forced vital capacity. Based on the Expert Panel report 3 of the National Heart, Lung, and Blood Institute (2007).

ASTHMA SEVERITY	SYMPTOMS	NIGHTTIME AWAKENING	USE OF SHORT ACTING BETA-2 AGONIST	INTERFERENCE WITH NORMAL ACTIVITY	LUNG FUNCTION
Intermittent	≤ 2 days/wk	≤ 2 days/mo	≤ 2 days/wk	None	Normal FEV1 between exacerbations FEV1 > 80% predicted FEV1/FVC normal
Mild persistent	> 2 days/wk but not daily	3-4 times/mo	> 2 days/wk but not daily and not >1 time in any day	Minor	FEV1 =>80% predicted FEV1/FVC normal
Moderate persistent	Daily	> 1x/wk but not nightly	Daily	Some	FEV1 = 60%-80% predicted FEV1/FVC= reduced 5%
Severe persistent	Throughout the day	Often 7 times/ wk	Several times/day	Extreme	FEV1 < 60% predicted FEV1/FVC reduced >5%

Chapter 9

Food Allergy

Food allergy results from an immune response to a specific food. Such a response may be IgE or non-IgE mediated.

A *food allergen* is a specific portion of the food that elicits an allergic reaction. Food allergens have been identified in many foods.

About 2-3.5 % of adults and 6% of infants/children have confirmed food allergies. The prevalence of food allergies is higher in those with preexisting allergies such as allergic rhinitis or atopic dermatitis.

COMMON FOOD ALLERGENS

Although theoretically, any food can elicit an IgE-mediated allergic reaction, only certain foods commonly do so. These, in decreasing order of prevalence, include milk, eggs, peanuts, tree nuts, shellfish, fish, wheat, and soy **(Fig. 9-1)**. The major allergens of common allergenic foods are depicted in **Figure 9-2**.

FIGURE 9-1. COMMON ALLERGENIC FOODS (IN DECREASING ORDER OF PREVALENCE)
Milk
Eggs
Peanuts
Tree nuts
Shellfish
Fish
Wheat
Soy

Milk is perhaps the most important source of nutrition in infants and children. Cow's milk consists of 90% water, 5% carbohydrates and 4-5% proteins. Milk allergy is a reaction to non-human milk such as cow's or goat's milk; therefore, infants or young children who are not breast-fed are at risk for an allergic reaction.

Milk proteins are grouped into casein and whey, either of which or both may cause an allergic reaction. The whey group proteins consist of *beta-lactoglobulin*, *alfa-lactalbumin*, and *serum albumin*. Milk allergy develops in the first year of life, but most allergic patients outgrow it by age 16 years.

Egg allergy is the second most common type of food allergy; it develops between 6-24 months of age.

Approximately 2/3 of patients outgrow egg allergy by the age of 16. *Egg white* contains 4 allergenic proteins: *ovomucoid* (Gal d1), *ovalbumin* (Gal d2), *ovotransferrin* (Gal d3), and *lysozyme* (Gal d4). In addition, two *egg yolk* allergens have been identified: *α-livetin* (chicken serum albumin, Gal d5) and *lipoprotein YGP 42* (Gal d6). Egg white has higher allergenic potential than egg yolk.

Peanuts are an important food allergen. Peanuts belong to the legume family. They are a known cause of food anaphylaxis. As of 2014, 13 peanut allergens have been identified, designated as *Ara h1* to *Ara h13*. Due to the nature of peanut hypersensitivity, i.e. anaphylaxis, studies on peanut allergy treatments have been limited. A presently ongoing study in the US uses a peanut patch to build immunotolerance in allergic patients. At present, the best strategy for prevention of an allergic reaction is avoidance.

There is cross-reactivity among *tree nuts*. Two examples are cashew/pistachio and walnut/pecan. In addition, there is cross-reactivity between tree nuts and peanuts.

Shellfish

Shellfish allergy is a major cause of food allergy in adults. This group consists of *crustaceans* (such as shrimp, lobster, prawn, crab and crawfish) and *mollusks* (such as clams, oysters and mussels). The food allergen in shrimp is a *tropomyosin* designated as *Pen a* 1.

Fish allergy is a reaction to the protein *parvalbumin*, found in the muscles of most fish. Fish is added to a number of food preparations, e.g. pizza toppings, some sausage, oyster sauce, Caesar salad, and surimi (imitation crab).

Wheat allergy. The prevalence of wheat allergy is about 0.4%. Approximately 2/3 of patients outgrow it by age 12. The allergen cross-reacts with rye, barley, oats and grasses. The allergic patient should be aware of this cross-reactivity and be cautious about unlabeled food. The wheat's protein (in seeds) consists of four classes:

1. *Albumins* (water-soluble)
2. *Globulins* (salt-soluble)
3. *Gliadins* (ethanol-soluble) and
4. *Glutenins* (urea-, detergent-, or KOH-soluble). All are potentially allergenic. Wheat gluten is a complex of gliadins and glutenins.

FIGURE 9-2. MAJOR FOOD ALLERGENS				
FOOD	**SCIENTIFIC NAME**	**MAJOR ALLERGEN**	**DESIGNATION**	**EXAMPLES OF WHERE ALLERGEN IS FOUND**
Milk (cow)	Bos Taurus	Casein Whey : (beta-lactoglobulin; alfa-lactalbumin serum albumin)	αs, b, a and k-casein Bos d5 Bos d4 Bos d6	Ice cream; cheese; cakes; cream cheese; yogurt; artificial butter flavor; curds; whey and whey products
Egg (chicken egg)	Gallus Gallus domesticus	Egg white: Ovomucoid Ovalbumin Ovotransferrin Lysozyme Egg yolk: α-livetin Lipoprotein YGp42	Gal d1 Gal d2 Gal d3 Gal d4 Gal d5 Gal d6	Cream puffs; frosting; ice cream; mayonnaise; pudding; souffles
Peanuts	Arachis hypogea	Vicilin Conglutin Gycinin	Ara h1 Ara h2 Ara h3 Note: As of 2014, 13 peanut proteins have been identified as allergenic (Ara h1 to Ara h13)	Peanut sauce; peanut syrup; goober peas; beer nuts
Tree nuts (e.g. cashew nut)	Anacardium occidentale	Vicilin-like protein	Ana o 1	Nut oil; nut extracts; pine nuts
Crustacean shellfish	Crustacea	Tropomyosin	Gad c1	All foods made with shellfish
Fish (e.g. halibut)	Hippoglossus hippoglossus	Paravalbumin	Gad c1	Imitation seafood; roe (fish eggs); caviar
Wheat	Triticum aestivum (common wheat)	Albumins Globulins Gliadins Glutenins (Gluten)		Bread, crackers; cookies; cakes; cereals; pasta Also: hotdogs, ice cream; candies, chocolate bars; biscuits
Soy (soybean)	Glycine max	Vicilin; legumin	Gly m1 to Gly m8	Soy milk; soy drink; soy sauce; tofu

Soy belongs to the legume family. Soy allergy is a result of reaction to proteins in seeds, including *vicilin* and *legumin*. Soy is widely used in food preparation and food products such as soy milk, soy sauce, and tofu. In addition, it is used as texturizer, emulsifier and protein filler.

In addition to food allergy from eating soy, the inhalation of soy powder can cause asthma-like symptoms.

Food Cross-Reactivity

Those with allergies to one food may experience an allergic reaction to other foods. This cross-reactivity is due to a homology of the allergens within foods. The closer the food groups are, the higher the chance of cross reactivity. For example, the cross-reactivity of cow's milk to goat's milk is over 90%, whereas the cross-reactivity of a legume, such as peanuts, to other legumes such as peas or lentils is 5%.

Cross-reactivity also exists between pollens and foods. For example, those with ragweed allergy have a 55% chance of reacting to apples, peaches or honeydew.

There is also cross-reactivity between certain fruits and latex. For instance, those with an allergy to banana, avocado, or kiwi have an 11% chance of reactivity to latex-containing products such as latex gloves (**Fig. 9-3**).

FIGURE 9-3. *EXAMPLES OF CROSS-REACTIVITY AMONG FOODS*

ALLERGIES TO	CROSS-REACTIVITY	RELATIVE COMPARISON
Cow's milk	Goat's milk	Very high
Cow's milk	Mare's milk	Low
Peanuts	Other legumes	Low
Peaches	Apples, pears	Moderate–high
Tree nuts	Other tree nuts	Moderate
Shellfish (e.g. shrimp)	Other shellfish: crab, lobster	High
Banana, avocado, kiwi	Latex	Low

Sometimes, allergic patients present with complaints of itching, swelling, hoarseness and discomfort in the oral cavity after ingesting a fresh fruit or vegetable. This phenomenon is known as *oral allergy syndrome*. It is due to cross-reactivity of food (fresh fruits and vegetables) and pollen allergens, which are homologous to the allergens in the particular fruit or vegetable. Interestingly, although the affected individuals experience the symptoms after ingesting fresh fruits and vegetables, they tolerate baked or cooked preparations well. The oral allergy syndrome is not rare; in fact, it is considered the most common food allergy in adults. Like other types of food allergies, the best prevention is to avoid ingesting the suspected fresh fruit and vegetables.

Food-dependent exercise-induced anaphylaxis is an interesting phenomenon in which two components (food and exercise) have to be present in order for the reaction to occur. In other words, the affected individual does not develop anaphylaxis with exercise or consumption of food alone. The typical scenario is an individual who ingests his meal containing wheat, celery, fish, or shellfish, and shortly later (2-4 hours) participates in some type of exercise regimen. The affected patient is usually atopic (has genetic predisposition). The best strategy to prevent such allergic reaction is to increase the time period between the meal and exercise.

Figure 9-4 lists the areas of the body affected by IgE-mediated reactions to food.

Figure 9-5 lists the immunologic spectrum of food adverse reactions and a few examples in each category

The *IgE-mediated food allergy* reaction is usually immediate, starting within a few minutes, but may also be delayed for a few hours. The sequence of events leading to the reaction is similar to reactions to aeroallergens (**Fig. 2-6**). The sequence starts with attachment of the a food-specific IgE to the high-affinity IgE receptor (FcεRI) on the surface of mast cells and basophils, resulting in their degranulation and release of inflammatory mediators. The

resulting reaction of vasodilation, smooth muscle contraction, mucus secretion, and microvascular leakage result from the actions of these mediators. Allergic reaction to food may be cutaneous (most common), pharyngeal, gastrointestinal, respiratory, cardiovascular, or neurological. One or multiple organ systems may be involved. The spectrum of reactions could range from cutaneous to systemic and life threatening (*anaphylaxis*)(**Figs. 9-4** and **9-5**).

FIGURE 9-4. *BODY AREAS AFFECTED BY IGE-MEDIATED FOOD REACTIONS*

ANATOMY INVOLVED	REACTIONS
Eyes	Pruritus; lacrimation
Nose	Rhinorrhea; nasal congestion
Ears	Pruritus
Oropharynx	Angioedema (lips, tongue); pruritus (palate)
Upper airway	Sneezing; stridor; laryngal edema; hoarseness
Lower airway	Cough; shortness of breath; wheezing
Gastrointestinal	Abdominal pain and cramping; bloating; nausea; vomiting; diarrhea
Cardiac	Tachycardia; arrhythmia; hypotension; cardiac arrest
Skin	Urticaria; angioedema; pruritus; flushing; morbilliform rash
Multiple organs	Anaphylaxis

Mixed IgE- and Non-IgE-Mediated Food Allergy

Atopic dermatitis. In populations of infants and young children with atopic dermatitis, approximately 33% have been shown to have food allergy reactions. The mechanism of the disease may be both IgE and non-IgE-mediated.

Eosinophilic esophagitis (EoE) is a chronic immune/antigen-mediated esophageal disease, characterized by the accumulation of eosinophils in esophageal tissues along with multiple subjective complaints and objective findings. The condition, while more common in infants and children, has also been diagnosed in adults. There is a spectrum of symptoms that starts in childhood and either changes or becomes less prevalent in adulthood. Two examples are food impaction, with a prevalence of 13% in pediatric patients and 51% in adults, and dysphagia in 30% of pediatric patients and 97% of adults.

Diagnosis of Eosinophilic Esophagitis (EoE)

Individuals with EoE are usually atopic. Therefore, the workup should include an allergy prick skin test for aero- and

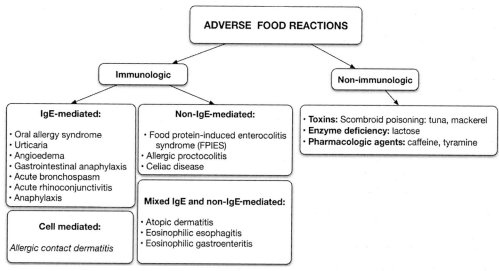

FIGURE 9-5. *Types of adverse food reactions.*

food allergens. In addition, lung function should be assessed with spirometry and/or a pulmonary function test for evaluation of possible asthma. The diagnosis of EoE is clinicopathologic. The microscopic presence of at least 15 eosinophils in a high power esophageal biopsy field is a pathological characteristic of EoE. In addition, EoE is characterized by certain unique histological, endoscopic, and radiographic features.

Histological characteristics of EoE include basal zone hyperplasia, superficial layering of surface eosinophils, eosinophilic microabscesses, dilated intercellular spaces, and subepithelial lamina propria fibrosis.

Endoscopic findings in EoE may include fixed or transient esophageal rings, whitish exudates (plaque), longitudinal furrows, diffuse esophageal narrowing, or edema.

Radiographic findings in EoE include concentric esophageal rings and narrowing.

Some patients may present with peripheral blood eosinophilia; this is a useful marker, as it correlates with tissue eosinophils and may be used for following the treatment success.

The only reliable diagnostic tests are endoscopy and biopsy.

In summary, the subjective complaints, along with the objective findings, collectively diagnose EoE.

Prevention/Treatment of Eosinophilic Esophagitis

1. *Avoid the offending food.* A combination of the subjective complaints and food prick skin testing can help to identify the offending food.

2. *Avoid solid, dry food.* There is always a potential risk of food impaction with certain foods such as steak or chicken, especially when they are dry.

3. *Chew food thoroughly* to prevent food impaction with larger pieces.

4. *Elemental formulas* are commercially prepared foods for children that contain elemental foods (amino acids). The logic is to use a simple and non-allergenic food. Some studies have shown significant resolution of symptoms and histological abnormalities with an elemental diet.

5. *Oral corticosteroids.* Systemic oral corticosteroids are considered an effective treatment of EoE; however, their side effects limit their long-term use.

6. *Topical corticosteroids* are effective and carry fewer side effects compared to oral corticosteroids. *Fluticasone* inhalers and *budesonide* (oral preparation for swallowing, not inhalation) are examples of commonly used corticosteroids.

DIAGNOSIS OF FOOD ALLERGY

History

History is an important part of the evaluation. In children, the information is provided by parents who have observed the food reactions. Affected adults may provide information about their food reactions, although sometimes the input from the spouse may be crucial. The clinician should ask pertinent questions to narrow the list of suspected foods:

1. Describe the food reaction? Was it a skin reaction (hives, swelling, or worsening eczema), a gastrointestinal reaction (nausea, vomiting, stomach cramps, or diarrhea)?

Comment: The type of reaction provides clues to the nature of the food reaction. For example, stomach cramps after ingesting dairy products is likely due to lactose intolerance.

2. Was this your first reaction? Or has it happened before?

Comment: The pattern of reactions gives a clue to the nature of the food in question. For example, if the reaction happens after a bad meal once, but never again with the same food, then suspect food poisoning.

3. How much food was consumed?

Comment: The true food allergic reaction results after ingesting a minute amount of the food. There are anecdotal reports of patients who claim that only large volumes of food cause the reaction; this history does not fit true food allergy.

4. Was the food raw or cooked?

Comment: This is important when oral allergy syndrome is suspected.

5. How did the reaction resolve? Did it resolve on its own or after medication?

Comment: This information is needed to assess the severity and persistence of the reaction.

Physical Examination

The physical exam consists of a general examination with emphasis on the eyes, face, oral cavity, nose, lungs, and skin.

Diagnostic Tests For Food Allergy

Prick skin test. The *prick skin* testing technique for food allergens resembles the test for aeroallergens. The upper back area of the patient is prepped with alcohol. The test area is marked with a marker and the allergens are pricked on the designated area one at a time. The results are interpreted after 15-20 minutes. Prick skin testing with food has high sensitivity and low specificity and therefore, positive results should be interpreted in correlation with clinical symptoms.

Intradermal test. Although the test is recommended for aeroallergens, it is not recommended for food allergens as it may cause an allergic reaction.

Patch test. The idea behind the patch test is that the food allergy may have a delayed reaction. This test has limited use and is not commonly performed. It consists of applying the food by a patch on the patient's upper back and interpreting the results 2 and 4 days post-application.

Food challenge. There are three types of food challenges: *open label*, *single blind*, and *double blind*. In an *open label* challenge, the patient and doctor are both aware of the tested food. In a *single blind* challenge, the patient alone is unaware (blind) of the tested allergen. In a *double blind test*, both patient and doctor are unaware of the tested food; the food allergen and a placebo are prepared by a third person. The blind challenge should be placebo-controlled for accuracy of diagnosis.

PREVENTION/TREATMENT OF FOOD ALLERGY

Unfortunately, there is no specific treatment for food allergy. Therefore, all the effort should be directed at prevention. Steps include:

1. Establish the diagnosis of food allergy by history, physical examination, and prick skin testing or by in-vitro IgE testing.

2. *Food Diary*. To help the diagnosis of food adverse reaction or allergy, the patient may keep a diary for recording food consumption and food reactions. The physician should review the food diary and look for a pattern of symptoms that correlates with a specific food.

3. *Food elimination*. The patient eliminates one food item at a time from his/her regular diet. If the symptom(s) persist, then he/she eliminates another item until the symptom(s) resolve. The suspected allergen can be identified by repeating the addition and elimination of the suspected food item from the diet.

4. *Read labels*. The Food Allergen Labeling Act and Consumer Protection Act (FALCPA) of 2004 (USA) requires that 8 food groups, considered "major food allergens," should be labeled. This guideline applies to food products that are labeled on or after January 1, 2006. The major food groups are milk, eggs, fish (e.g. bass, flounder, cod), shellfish (e.g. crab, lobster, shrimp), tree nuts (e.g. almonds, walnuts, pecans), peanuts, wheat, and soybeans.

5. Avoid the known or suspicious food allergen.

6. Watch for *cross-contamination*. Say you have a fish allergy and order a fish-free meal in a restaurant. The next table in the restaurant orders fish. After preparing the fish meal for the adjacent table, the cook uses the same pan and prepares your meal that is supposedly fish-free. After ingesting your meal you develop hives, even though you are not consuming fish. What happened was cross-contamination of the fish allergen fish previously made in the same pan with your meal. This reaction can be prevented by washing the pan thoroughly after each meal preparation, or by designating separate cookware for each food group.

7. *Breastfeeding for ages 4-6 months*. This is important to reduce the risk of cow's milk allergy.

8. Be prepared to treat allergic reactions, specifically anaphylaxis. Patients should carry injectable epinephrine.

Chapter 10
Drug Allergy

Adverse Drug Reactions (ADRs) are divided into two major categories, Type A and Type B.

TYPE A DRUG REACTIONS (DOSE-DEPENDENT)

The *Type A* reaction comprises an estimated 85-90% of all ADRs. This class, which occurs in healthy individuals, is predictable from the known *dose-dependent* pharmacological properties of the drug. Some examples include dry mouth due to diphenhydramine (an antihistamine) and nausea with codeine. Drug overdose, drug side effects, and drug interactions are also included in this category (**Fig. 10-1**).

TYPE B DRUG REACTIONS (DOSE-INDEPENDENT)

Type B reactions comprise about 10-15% of all ADRs. This class is unpredictable and *dose-independent*. An example is anaphylaxis due to penicillin. Type B ADRs are further divided into drug intolerance, drug idiosyncrasy, and immunogenic (drug allergy and drug pseudoallergy) types:

- *Drug Intolerance.* This unpredictable type of reaction may occur with a low or a regular dose of a medication (e.g. aspirin-induced tinnitus).

- *Drug Idiosyncrasy.* This type of ADR is genetically determined and is related to a metabolic or enzyme deficiency. An example is hemolytic anemia after primaquin therapy in a patient with G6PD deficiency. Some drugs cause idiosyncratic toxicities. Examples are rhabdomyolysis and liver toxicity due to antipsychotic drugs such as chlorpromazine.

- *Immunogenic Drug Reaction (drug allergy).* Based on Gell and Coombs classification, drug allergy may be of the Type I, Type II, Type III or Type IV variety (**Fig. 2-1**). Long after the Gell and Coombs classification was introduced, a modification of Type IV hypersensitivity was proposed that divides Type IV hypersensitivity into four subtypes, IV a-d. This classi-

TYPE	CAUSE	REACTION PREDICTABLLITY	DOSE DEPENDENCY	EXAMPLES
Type A (Dose dependent)	Overdose, side effects, drug interaction	+	+	• Hepatic failure (acetaminophen overdose) • Dry mouth (diphenhdyramine) • QT prolongation (erythroycin and quinidine drug interaction)
Type B (Dose independent)	Intolerance	−	−	Aspirin-induced tinnitus (Intolerance)
	Idiosyncrasy			Hemolytic anemia with primaquin in a patient with G6PD deficiency (Idiosyncrasy)
	Immunogenic: Type I Hypersensitivity Type II Hypersensitivity Type III Hypersensitivity Type IV Hypersensitivity (subtypes IV a-d)			• Urticaria; anaphylaxis due to penicillin (Type I) • Penicillin-induced hemolytic anemia and thrombocytopenia (Type II) • Serum sickness (Type III) • Contact dermatitis to neomycin (Type IV)

FIGURE 10-1. CLASSIFICATION 0F ADVERSE DRUG REACTIONS

fication recognizes activation and recruitment of macrophages (Type IVa), eosinophils (Type IVb), T cells (Type IVc), and neutrophils (Type IVd).

Pseudoallergy

Pseudoallergy refers to an allergy-like reaction to a substance, such as drug, that does not fit the Gell and Coombs classification; although these reactions mimic the immunologic type reactions in appearance, their exact underlying mechanisms have not been confirmed. Some examples of drugs causing pseudoallergic reactions include:

1. *Vancomycin.* Vancomycin may induce an IgE-mediated anaphylaxis or a non-IgE-mediated "pseudoallergic" reaction (*Redman Syndrome*), which results from rapid infusion of the medication, leading to degranulation of mast cells and release of histamine. The patient usually experiences pruritus, erythematous rash, and diffuse burning. The reactions commonly involve the face, neck and upper torso. Pre-medication with an H1 receptor blocker antihistamine, such as diphenhydramine, and slowing the vancomycin infusion rate (1 gram/hour) help to prevent the reaction.

2. *Aspirin and Non-Steroid Anti-Inflammatory Drugs (NSAIDs).* Aspirin and NSAIDs act by blocking the cyclooxygenase-1 (COX-1) enzyme, resulting in inhibition of prostaglandin synthesis. This class of medication can cause urticaria, angioedema, and anaphylaxis, and exacerbate underlying respiratory disease such as asthma. In addition, the reaction to this class of medication may also be IgE-mediated. Patients, whether "allergic" or "pseudoallergic," should avoid aspirin and all NSAID preparations.

3. *Radiocontrast Media (RCM).* Some people experience an anaphylactoid reaction after receiving radiocontrast media. There is a "myth" that patients with seafood allergy are at greater risk of developing anaphylaxis than the general population; however, this relationship has not been substantiated. Certain people are at greater risk of reaction to RCM. These are individuals who have had prior reactions to RCM, a history of cardiovascular disease or asthma, and those on beta blocker medication. Replacing RCM with a non-ionic contrast media, and premedication with diphenhydramine and prednisone, can reduce the chance of an anaphylactoid reaction.

4. *Opiates.* Opiates can directly induce mast cells and basophils to degranulate. The release of histamine causes pruritus and urticaria.

DIAGNOSIS OF DRUG ALLERGY

History

The following are key questions when assessing for a patient's drug allergy:

1. What type of reaction have you experienced? Hives (urticaria), swelling (angioedema), closing throat (laryngioedema), or systemic symptoms (anaphylaxis)?

Comment: This information helps us to understand the severity of the reaction and prepare the patient for future incidents.

2. Was this your first experience with this medication?
3. Can you identify which one of your medications caused your symptoms?
4. How did you take your medication? Was it on an empty stomach? With food? Did you follow the directions on how to take the medication? Did you follow the dosage instruction?
5. If you do not know the name of your medication, can you bring the bottle with you on the next visit?
6. What other medications do you take?

Comment: The above information helps us to check for drug interactions and to assess the possibility of cross-reactivity, for drug allergy, or synergistic effects of multiple drugs.

Prick Skin Test for Sensitivity

The IgE-mediated test can be performed by prick skin testing. Briefly, the drug in question is administered by pricking the skin and looking for an inflammatory reaction within about 30 minutes. The test should be validated with a negative control, such as saline (salt water) and a positive control, such as histamine. A negative test can be followed by an intradermal test.

With the exception of a test for penicillin allergy, there is no other standardized in-vivo drug testing available on the market. Penicillin testing is an important test that can largely exclude a penicillin allergy. Thousands of people are labeled with "penicillin allergy." However, they are mostly unable to recall the nature of this "allergy." The majority of these patients remotely remember their parents telling them they are allergic to penicillin. Since penicillin is still the drug of choice for many infections, investigation to substantiate the nature of this supposed allergy is important and life saving in many instances.

The subject should be tested with major and minor penicillin determinant allergens. (*Antigen determinant* refers to the site on the surface of an antigen molecule to which the antibody binds. This is a site that determines the immunologic specificity). Reportedly, the negative predictive value for an immediate reaction is close to 100% and the positive predictive value of the test is 40-100%.

Patients with a history of penicillin allergy who need to receive cephalosporins should be tested for penicillin allergy, because of cross-reactivity of cephalosporin and penicillin. If the test with major and minor determinants is negative, then there is minimal concern about an immediate IgE-mediated reaction with cephalosporin.

Test Dosing (Graded Challenge)

The dose testing of a drug consists of administering increasing increments of the drug until reaching the full dose. The goal of the test is to identify individuals with immediate adverse reactions.

Patch Testing

Patch testing identifies the delayed reaction to a drug. The test is intended to identify allergic contact dermatitis to a medication. The test consists of applying a patch embedded with the drug of interest, such as neomycin, to the patient's upper back. The patch is removed after 48 hours (first reading) and the area is observed for another 48 hours for final interpretation. A positive test is an area of redness with or without induration (based on severity) (**Fig. 7-2**).

Tips to Avoid Drug Allergy

- Educate the patient not to take unknown medications.
- Check the drug interactions.
- A thorough history can help assess the nature of the drug allergy.
- Test a new drug with a questionable history of "drug allergy."
- Monitor the patient after administering the drug in question.
- Write the words "drug allergy to. . ." on the chart.
- Avoid administering the same medication.
- Recommend to the patient a drug allergy identifier such as a bracelet or a necklace,
- Change the allergenic drug to an alternative medication if possible.

TREATMENT OF DRUG SENSITIVITY

A problem arises when a patient has multiple drug allergies and it is difficult to find a substitute medication. Then the last option is *drug desensitization*. The broader term to describe this phenomenon is *induction of drug tolerance*. This is a procedure that involves an introduction of a low dose of the drug in question (in microgram range) followed by stepwise administration of higher doses to a full dose. The goal is to ensure that the patient can tolerate the full dose of a drug without an adverse reaction. Sensitization is a temporary solution for tolerating a drug allergy (**Fig. 10-2**). In other words the sensitivity is short-lived and lasts for the duration in which the patient takes the medication. The advantage of drug desensitization is that after completing the desensitization protocol the patient is able to take the drug safely, without adverse reaction.

FIGURE 10-2. INDICATIONS FOR DRUG DESENSITIZATION	
INDICATIONS	**COMMENT**
When the allergic medication is the drug of choice	The drug of choice is backed up with studies and the efficacy of the treatment is established. An example is use of sulfamethoxazole-trimethoprim for treatment of *Pneumocystis jiroveci* pneumonia.
Multiple drug allergies	There are no choices to treat with similar medication due to multiple drug allergies.
When the treatment with non-allergic drugs has failed	Other non-allergic medications were tried and failed.
Unavailability of similarly effective drug	At times the medication may be the only effective drug or the only available drug. For example, omalizumab is the only anti-IgE medication on the US market.
Proof of successful treatment in the literature	Various desensitization protocols are available in the literature. Examples are sulfamethoxazole-trimethoprim, aspirin, and penicillin.

The disadvantage of drug desensitization is that after completing the desensitization protocol the patient should continue taking the medication on a regular basis; by stopping the medication, the patient loses the sensitization and again becomes sensitized to the drug. In other words, desensitization is a temporary means of tolerating the drug; if the patient needs the same medication in the future, this requires another round of desensitization protocol.

Fig. 10-3 summarizes the management of drug reaction.

EVALUATION OF DRUG REACTIONS

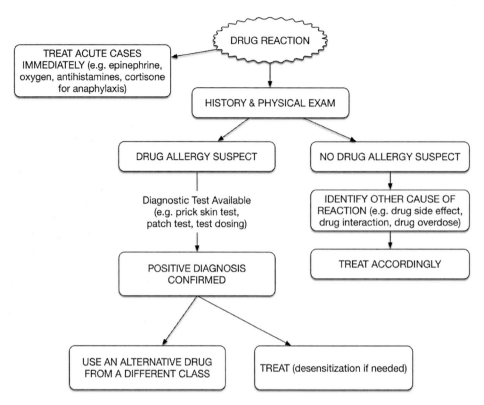

FIGURE 10-3.

Chapter 11
Immunotherapy

Immunotherapy is a treatment regimen that renders an allergic patient immune to the harm of a specific allergen. Although the term *desensitization* has been used, the more accurate terminology is *allergy immunotherapy* or *allergy vaccination*. The technique consists of administration of increasing dose of antigen(s) into the host in identical time intervals. The time period in which the dose of antigen is increasing is known as the "build-up phase." The allergens are injected subcutaneously once or twice a week. In approximately 4-8 months (depending on frequency of injections, once or twice a week), the injecting allergen dose is no longer increased and the host starts receiving the same dose; this time period is known as the "maintenance phase." For the remaining period of immunotherapy, the host receives the same dose of allergen in identical intervals.

Allergy immunotherapy is indicated for allergic rhinitis, allergic rhinoconjunctivitis, allergic asthma, and venom allergies. In addition, allergy immunotherapy may benefit a subgroup of patients who have atopic dermatitis and pollen allergy.

There is no indication for immunotherapy in treating urticaria, angioedema, allergic contact dermatitis, or food or latex allergy. However several trials for peanuts and wheat are in progress, but since the final outcome of the studies are unavailable at the time of this writing, immune therapy for food allergy is considered experimental (**Fig. 11-1**).

FIGURE 11-1. INDICATIONS & NON-INDICATIONS FOR IMMUNOTHERAPY	
INDICATIONS	**NON-INDICATIONS**
Allergic rhinitis	Urticaria
Allergic rhinoconjunctivitis	Angioedema
Allergic asthma	Allergic contact dermatitis
Venom allergies (anaphylaxis)	Food allergy
Some patients with atopic dermatitis	Latex allergy

HOW DOES IMMUNOTHERAPY WORK? PATHOPHYSIOLOGY

After starting immunotherapy, the immune system undergoes a series of complex immunological reactions, some of which are still unknown.

One of the important immune responses to immunotherapy is reduction of the specific IgE. After initiation of immunotherapy there is a surge of the IgE, which may or may not correlate with increasing clinical symptoms, followed by a gradual fall of IgE production. Another response to immunotherapy is production of specific IgGs known as *blocking antibodies*. It is hypothesized that these blocking antibodies compete with the IgE binding to the allergens. As a result, the allergen-induced IgE-dependent mast calls and basophils are inhibited. There is also evidence that these blocking antibodies inhibit allergen-IgE binding to B cells, a step in antigen presentation to T cells. The surge of IgG blocking antibodies does not necessarily correlate with improvement of symptoms.

A simplistic way of demonstrating this relationship is depicted in **Figure 11-2**. The actual response curve to immunotherapy varies, depending on the allergen and the degree of immune response.

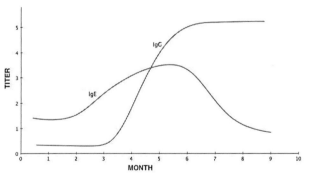

FIGURE 11-2. IgE and IgG levels in immunotherapy.

As noted earlier (See **Fig. 2-6**), Th2 cells participate in Type I hypersensitivity. Atopic patients favor formation of Th2, thereby promoting hypersensitivity, whereas non-allergic patients favor formation of Th1. Formation of Th1 or Th2 depends on participation of various regulatory factors as depicted in **Figure 11-3**. One of the outcomes of immunotherapy is a shift of Th2 pathway to the Th1 pathway.

And finally, successful immunotherapy leads to reduction of early and late phase allergy responses to allergens.

TH1 / TH2 BALANCE

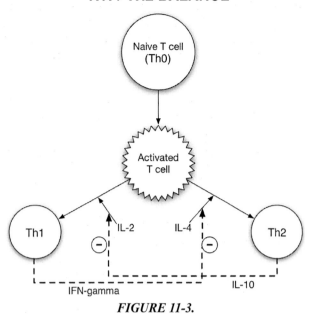

FIGURE 11-3.

TYPES OF IMMUNOTHERAPY

There are several types of immunotherapy, based on route of administration:

1. *Nasal Allergy Immunotherapy (Local Nasal Immunotherapy, LNIT).* This type of immunotherapy involves administering allergens nasally. This helps for allergic rhinitis, as shown in many randomized double-blind placebo-controlled studies. The advantage of this therapy is convenience of self-administration and cost-effectiveness, as the patient saves frequent trips to the health provider for the allergen administrations. The disadvantage is that the patient needs to follow a specific technique to ensure delivery of the allergen effectively (**Fig. 11-4**).

2. *Subcutaneous Allergen Immunotherapy (SCIT).* This type of immunotherapy involves administration of the allergens subcutaneously. It is the most common type of immunotherapy, is backed by many controlled studies, and has been successfully used worldwide. The advantage of this method of therapy is its effectiveness, safety, and ease of administration. However, the time spent to go the doctor's office for administering the allergen and the waiting period after each injection is limiting for some (**Fig 11-4**).

3. *Sublingual Immunotherapy (SLIT).* This form of immunotherapy has more recently been approved by the Food and Drug Administration (FDA) and has entered the US market. Its advantage is ease of administration, since the patient can take the prescribed medication

FIGURE 11-4. TYPES OF ALLERGY IMMUNOTHERAPY						
TYPE OF IMMUNO-THERAPY	**ROUTE OF ADMINIS-TRATION**	**EFFEC-TIVENESS**	**SAFETY**	**ADVANTAGES**	**DISADVAN-TAGES**	**NOTE**
Nasal Immunotherapy	Nasal	+	+	Ease of administration; fewer doctor visits; cost effective	Specific administration technique needed; used only for allergic rhinitis	Not available in the U.S.
Subcutaneous Immunotherapy (SCIT)	Skin (subcutaneous)	+	+	Ease of administration; effectiveness	Injections have to be in health provider's office; time spent for injections (commuting to the office and a waiting period post-injection)	Most commonly utilized method of immunotherapy worldwide
Sublingual Immunotherapy (SLIT)	Oral (sublingual)	+	+	Dec chance of anaphylaxis; ease of self-administration; no need to see a doctor for administration; time saver		

outside the doctor's office. It has been proven safe, with minimal adverse reaction. However, due to limited availability of the allergenic products, its use is presently limited (**Fig. 11-4**).

WHO IS A CANDIDATE FOR IMMUNOTHERAPY (FIG. 11-5)?

Candidates for immunotherapy include:

- *Patients with moderate to severe symptoms.* The symptoms are unbearable and medications are not sufficient to control the symptoms.
- *Patients with prolonged symptoms.* The symptoms are persistent and frequent. An example is daily, year-round symptoms due to dust mite allergy.
- *Patients with medication side effects.* Sometimes, patients cannot tolerate the medication. They may experience discomfort or irritation (e.g. nasal irritation after a nasal spray or burning eyes after use of an ophthalmic antihistamine).
- *Failure of medication.* The medications may fail to resolve the symptoms, and the patient seeks an alternative therapy. The only other alternative to preventive measures and medication may be immunotherapy. Looking at the bigger picture, environmental protection measures and medications are just temporary means of allergy management; however, immunotherapy is a cure.

Adherence to the long course of immunotherapy is a commitment for the duration of the therapy. Therefore, the patient should understand the procedure, the range of outcomes, and possible side effects, and be determined to complete the course of treatment. There is no indication for immunotherapy if the symptoms are mild and last a few weeks of the year. The mild symptoms may be managed by taking antihistamines (oral, nasal, or ophthalmic). When the symptoms last more than a few weeks, like the whole season or more than one season, then immunotherapy may be the best option.

- *Anaphylaxis due to venom.* Venom immunotherapy is the only effective way of preventing anaphylaxis due to venom stings.
- *Patient's choice.* Some patients dislike using nasal sprays or oral medication due to irritation (nasal sprays) and other side effects (oral medications).

Selecting Allergens for Immunotherapy (Figs. 11-6 and 11-7)

The decision to select appropriate allergens for immunotherapy in symptomatic patients is based on the intensity of the skin reactions. The size of the reaction on skin testing is compared with the reaction from the positive control sample, which consists of histamine. Then, the allergens with the same or bigger reaction than the positive control are chosen for immunotherapy.

Allergen Dilutions

After selecting allergens for the therapy, they are mixed in a sterile fashion. There are different ways of mixing the allergens. One way is to mix them in a ratio of 1:1, e.g. mixing 0.5 ml of a selected allergen with 0.5 ml of another allergen. This is considered the "stock bottle," which contains a mixture of the desired allergens for the therapy. The stock bottle is then diluted 1:10; this can be done simply by taking 0.5 ml of the reagent and adding it to 4.5 ml of diluent. (Each bottle of diluent contains pre-measured 4.5 ml of saline solution.) The next dilutions are done the same way,

FIGURE 11-5. CRITERIA OF PATIENT SELECTION FOR IMMUNOTHERAPY	
CRITERIA	**NOTE**
Moderate to severe symptoms	This is when the symptoms are unbearable and medication is not sufficient to control them.
Prolonged symptoms	This is when the symptoms are persistent and frequent. An example is daily, year-round symptoms due to dust mite allergy.
Medication side effects/ adverse reactions	Discomfort or irritation (e.g. nasal irritation after a nasal spray or burning eyes after use of an ophthalmic antihistamine).
Medication failure	Tachyphylaxis (diminishing efficacy of a medication) or medication ineffectiveness points toward immunotherapy.
Anaphylaxis	This is specific to venom allergens.
Patient's choice	Various personal reasons may result in choosing immunotherapy

FIGURE 11-6. PRESCRIPTIONS FOR ORAL IMMUNOTHERAPY					
FDA: Food and Drug Administration; IR= Index of reactivity; BAU: Bioavailability Unit Category B: Animal reproduction studies have failed to demonstrate a risk to the fetus but there are no adequate and well-controlled studies in pregnant women. Category C: Animal reproduction studies *have* shown an adverse effect on the fetus, but there are no adequate and well-controlled studies in humans. Potential benefits, though, may warrant use of the drug in pregnant women despite risks under certain circumstances.					
DRUG	**AGE (YRS) OF ADMINISTRATION**	**DAY 1**	**DAY 2**	**DAY 3 AND BEYOND**	**NOTE**
Oralair	Under 10 and over 65				Not approved by FDA
	10-17	100 IR	2x 100 IR	300 IR	Pregnancy Category B
	18-65	300 IR	300 IR	300 IR	
Grastek	Under 5 and over 65				Not approved by FDA
	5-65	2800 BAU	Same as day 1	Same as day 1	Pregnancy Category B
Ragwitek	Under 18 and over 65				Not approved by FDA
	18-65	12 Amb a 1-unit (Amb a 1-U)	Same as day 1	Same as day 1	Pregnancy Category C

FIGURE 11-7. AVAILABLE ALLERGENS FOR ORAL IMMUNOTHERAPY IN THE US MARKET			
ALLERGENS	**AVAILABLE IN US**	**BRAND NAME**	**AGE INDICATION**
Grass	Five-pollen combination: sweet vernal; orchard; perennial rye; timothy; Kentucky blue grass	Oralair	10 to 65 years
	Timothy	Grastek	5 to 65 years
Weeds	Short ragweed	Ragwitek	18 to 65 years

making 1:100, 1:1000, 1:10,000, and 1:100,000 preparation bottles (**Figure 11-8**).

Phases of Immunotherapy

There are two phases of immunotherapy: the *buildup phase* and the *maintenance phase*. The buildup phase refers to the duration of time in which the treatment dose is increasing. The ultimate dose after which the treatment dose stays the same is called the *maintenance dose*. The maintenance phase is the duration of time in which the patient receives the maintenance dose (**Fig. 11-9**).

Allergy Immunotherapy Schedule

The therapy starts with injecting a low dose allergen mixture from the most diluted bottle. For patients with severe symptoms or when therapy starts during "problematic season," the 1:100,000 bottle is a safe dilution to start. Otherwise choosing from the 1:10,000 dilution bottle can be designated as the starting dose.

The injections are administered once or twice a week. As the dose increases, i.e. it becomes more concentrated, weekly injections are preferred. The decision to select the

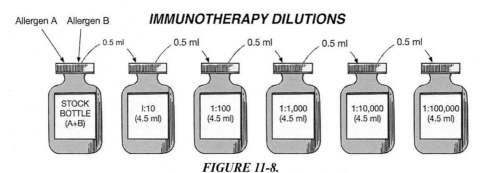

IMMUNOTHERAPY DILUTIONS

FIGURE 11-8.

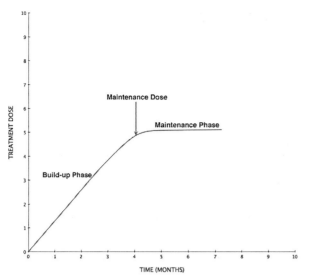

FIGURE 11-9. Dosage phases in immunotherapy.

immunotherapy doses varies among allergists. The goal is to reach the 0.5 ml dose of the 1:100 dilution bottle; this is considered the maintenance dose. However, **Figure 11-10** is simply an example schedule, as the response to immunotherapy varies among individuals due to their sensitivity to the allergen extract. Therefore the decision to choose the maintenance dose should be individualized. One factor in selecting the dose is the local reaction at the injection dose (early and delayed response) and the general response to the treatment dose. For instance, if the patient has a larger than 1-2 centimeter diameter erythema/induration at the site of injection, caution must be exercised when increasing the treatment dose.

One expects to see at least some local reaction at the site of injection, especially in higher treatment doses. If there is no reaction even with the maintenance dose, the allergist needs to review the results of skin testing and the allergen mixture preparation for any signs of error. If all the reagents were mixed as planned and no error in treatment mixture is detected, then one option is to increase the dose by using a more concentrated treatment bottle, 1:10 dilution, or stop the treatment and consider it ineffective.

Duration of Immunotherapy

The recommendation for a complete course of immunotherapy is 3-5 years. However, the decision to stop the treatment should be individualized. The following are examples of factors that direct the duration of immunotherapy:

* *The patient did not follow the regular scheduled regimen* and received the injections irregularly. For example, if one dose of weekly injection was missed,

then the allergist may choose not to increase the dose; this places the patient one week behind schedule. If two doses (two weeks of injections) were missed, then the allergist may reduce the dose; for example if the patient, while on a weekly schedule, received 0.1 ml of the 1:100 dilution and missed two weekly doses, then the allergist may administer 0.05 ml of the 1:100 as opposed to increasing the dose to 0.15 ml; this places the patient two weeks behind schedule. The patient who continues attending the scheduled injections irregularly may need to continue treatment beyond the customary 3-5 years of therapy.

* *Ineffective therapy* is a reason to terminate the treatment. The treatment for those who are at their maintenance dose of treatment and are still symptomatic should be re-evaluated. One option is to increase the dose, if possible; the only other option is to terminate the treatment. It usually takes about a year from start of the immunotherapy to confirm the ineffectiveness of the treatment.

* *Repeated anaphylaxis* is a reason to stop the treatment; this is especially true when the cause of anaphylaxis is idiopathic.

* *Patient's choice* is a factor in determining the length of therapy. There are patients who benefit from the therapy only a short time after stopping the scheduled course of treatment. For this subgroup of patients, the treatment may continue beyond the recommended customary course of therapy. In other words, this subgroup of patients loses their immune tolerance to the specific allergens sooner than expected.

Note than allergy immunotherapy and drug desensitization are two separate topics. Immunotherapy can be a cure, but drug desensitization is not and is only temporary. For drug desensitization the patient must continue exposure to the drug after the desensitization protocol or the adverse response will recur.

There are two options regarding the length of venom therapy. One option is to continue the treatment for 3-5 years. The other option is to continue it, depending on the level of IgE. For example, if the patient receiving treatment for yellow jacket venom is retested after 3-5 years and does not have detectable yellow jacket IgE, then the therapy can be terminated; otherwise, the allergist may choose to continue the therapy beyond the customary period.

The effect of immunotherapy can last for years, up to a lifetime. However, the duration of immunity may be shortened for various reasons, including continuous exposure to the allergens, illness, new medications, moving to a new environment with higher surrounding allergens, and, finally, aging.

FIGURE 11-10. IMMUNOTHERAPY TREATMENT SCHEDULE					
ALLERGEN	**1:100,000**	**1:10,000**	**1:1000**	**1:100**	**COMMENT**
Week 1	0.05 ml	(ml)	(ml)	(ml)	Bottle #1
Week 2	0.1 ml				
Week 3	0.2 ml				
Week 4	0.3 ml				
Week 5	0.4 ml				
Week 6	0.5 ml				
Week 7		0.05 ml			Bottle #2
Week 8		0.1 ml			
Week 9		0.2 ml			
Week 10		0.3 ml			
Week 11		0.4 ml			
Week 12		0.5 ml			
Week 13			.05 ml		Bottle #3
Week 14			0.1 ml		
Week 15			0.15 ml		
Week 16			0.2 ml		
Week 17			0.25 ml		
Week 18			0.3 ml		
Week 19			0.35 ml		
Week 20			0.4 ml		
Week 21			0.45 ml		
Week 22			0.5 ml		
Week 23				0.05 ml	Bottle #4
Week 24				0.1 ml	
Week 25				0.15 ml	
Week 26				0.2 ml	
Week 27				0.25 ml	
Week 28				0.3 ml	
Week 29				0.35 ml	
Week 30				0.4 ml	
Week 31				0.45 ml	
Week 32				0.5 ml	Maintenance Dose
Week 33-36				0.5 ml	Once/wk
Week 37-45				0.5 ml	Every 2 wks
Week 46-58				0.5 ml	Every 3 wks
Week 59 +				0.5 ml	Every 4 wks until course completion

APPENDIX

ALLERGY QUESTIONNAIRE

1. Are your symptoms seasonal? ❑ Yes ❑ No If yes, which season is your worst one? ❑ Fall ❑ Winter ❑ Spring ❑ Summer?
2. Are your symptoms all year-round (perennial)? ❑ Yes ❑ No
3. Are your symptoms year-round but worsen in a certain season? ❑ Yes ❑ No
   If so, what season? ❑ Fall ❑ Winter ❑ Spring ❑ Summer
4. How long have you had the symptoms?
   ❑ This year only ❑ Over a year ❑ Since I moved to the area
5. Specifically, have you had your symptoms since:
   ❑ Childhood? ❑ Teenage years? ❑ Adulthood?
6. What do you do or have you done to control your symptoms?
   ❑ Medication ❑ Other Please explain_____

   _____
7. How bad are your symptoms? ❑ Just annoying ❑ Debilitating
   Do you miss school or work days? ❑ Yes ❑ No
   Do you visit a doctor or an emergency room for flare-ups? ❑ Yes ❑ No
8. Does medication control your symptoms?
   ❑ Yes ❑ Just for few hours ❑ Not at all
9. What are your symptoms? ❑ Nasal ❑ Eyes ❑ Respiratory
10. How is your sense of taste or smell? ❑ Good ❑ Poor ❑ None
11. Are you a mouth breather or a nose breather? ❑ Mouth ❑ Nose
12 What triggers your symptoms?
   ❑ Dust ❑ Pet exposure ❑ Pollen ❑ Cold weather ❑ Heat ❑ Other Explain_____

   _____
13. Do you use any over-the-counter nasal sprays or eye drops such as those containing phenylephrine or oxymetazoline?
   ❑ No ❑ Sometimes ❑ Regularly
14. Are you currently taking any antihistamine, oral, nasal, or ophthalmic?
   ❑ Nasal spray ❑ Eye drops ❑ Oral medication
15. If you do not take any antihistamine, is it because of:
   ❑ Medication failure ❑ Side effects ❑ Cost ❑ Personal choice
16. How often do you take your medication(s)?
   ❑ Daily ❑ During my season ❑ A few days at a time
17. Do you get sinus infections? ❑ Yes ❑ No If so, how often?_____

   _____
18. Have you ever had pneumonia? ❑ Yes ❑ No
   If so, does it occur more than 4-5 times a year? ❑ Yes ❑ No
19. Do you have asthma? ❑ Yes ❑ No
20. Have you had any nasal surgery? ❑ Yes ❑ No
   If so, what type of surgery? ❑ Nasal fracture ❑ Turbinoplasty (reduction of turbinate bones) ❑ Septoplasty ❑ Polypectomy (removal of nasal polyps)
21. Have you had any operation in the ears such as ear tubes? ❑ Yes ❑ No
   If Yes, how many times?_____
22. Do any of your immediate family members (parents, siblings or children) have allergies? ❑ Yes ❑ No If so, who?_____

   _____

Home Environment

23. Where do you live?
    ❏ In town ❏ Downtown ❏ Close to freeway ❏ Suburbs ❏ Mountains
24. What kind of building do you live in? ❏ House ❏ Apartment ❏ Duplex
25. How old is the building?_____
26. How many levels is your residence?____ Is it a single floor? ❏ Yes ❏ No
    Describe_____
27. Do you have a basement? ❏ Yes ❏ No If Yes, Is it damp? ❏ Yes ❏ No Does it flood in rain? ❏ Yes ❏ No
    Do you live in the basement? ❏ Yes ❏ No
28. What type of heater do you use at home?
    ❏ Central ❏ Furnace ❏ Fireplace
29. What type of cooling system do you use?
    ❏ Central ❏ Window unit ❏ Fan
30. If you have windows, are they ❏ Sealed ❏ Can be opened? How often do you open your windows?_____
31. What type of flooring do you have? ❏ Carpet ❏ Hardwood ❏ Tile ❏ Other
    Describe_____
32. What type of bedding do you have?
    ❏ Mattress only ❏ Mattress over a box spring
33. What material is your blanket, pillow, or mattress? ❏ Feather ❏ Synthetic
    Describe_____
34. What type of furniture do you have?
    ❏ Leather ❏ Vinyl ❏ Wood ❏ Upholstered
35. Do you have an aquarium? ❏ Yes ❏ No
36. Do you have pets? ❏ Yes ❏ No If yes, how many?____ What kind of pet(s)?_____

    _____
    Indoor or outdoor pets? ❏ Indoor ❏ Outdoor_____

    _____
    Do they come to your bedroom? ❏ Yes ❏ No
    Do you sleep with your pet(s) at night? ❏ Yes ❏ No

Work Environment (Answer if you work outside your home)

37. What type of building do you work in?
    ❏ Office building ❏ Warehouse
38. What type of air-conditioning or heating system do you have at work?
    ❏ Central ❏ Window unit ❏ Furnace
39. What type of flooring do you have at work?_____

    _____
40. Do you have windows at work? ❏ Yes ❏ No
    If so, are they ❏ Sealed ❏ Can be opened
41. How many employees work in the same room?
    ❏ Work alone ❏ 2-5 ❏ More than 5
42. Do you work in a ❏ Cubicle ❏ Your own room? How many cubicles are in the room? _____

    _____
    If you work in a cubicle, is it padded like upholstered material? ❏ Yes ❏ No
43. Do co-workers bring pets to work? ❏ Yes ❏ No

INDEX

RAPID LEARNING AND RETENTION THROUGH THE MEDMASTER SERIES:

CLINICAL NEUROANATOMY MADE RIDICULOUSLY SIMPLE, by S. Goldberg
CLINICAL BIOCHEMISTRY MADE RIDICULOUSLY SIMPLE, by S. Goldberg
CLINICAL ANATOMY MADE RIDICULOUSLY SIMPLE, by S. Goldberg and H. Ouellette
CLINICAL PHYSIOLOGY MADE RIDICULOUSLY SIMPLE, by S. Goldberg
CLINICAL MICROBIOLOGY MADE RIDICULOUSLY SIMPLE, by M. Gladwin, B. Trattler and C.S. Mahan
CLINICAL PHARMACOLOGY MADE RIDICULOUSLY SIMPLE, by J.M. Olson
OPHTHALMOLOGY MADE RIDICULOUSLY SIMPLE, by S. Goldberg
PSYCHIATRY MADE RIDICULOUSLY SIMPLE, by J. Nelson, W. Good and M. Ascher
CLINICAL PSYCHOPHARMACOLOGY MADE RIDICULOUSLY SIMPLE, by J. Preston and J. Johnson
USMLE STEP 1 MADE RIDICULOUSLY SIMPLE, by A. Carl
USMLE STEP 2 MADE RIDICULOUSLY SIMPLE, by A. Carl
USMLE STEP 3 MADE RIDICULOUSLY SIMPLE, by A. Carl
BEHAVIORAL MEDICINE MADE RIDICULOUSLY SIMPLE, by F. Seitz and J. Carr
ACID-BASE, FLUIDS, AND ELECTROLYTES MADE RIDICULOUSLY SIMPLE, by R. Preston
THE FOUR-MINUTE NEUROLOGIC EXAM, by S. Goldberg
MEDICAL SPANISH MADE RIDICULOUSLY SIMPLE, by T. Espinoza-Abrams
CLINICAL ANATOMY AND PHYSIOLOGY FOR THE ANGRY HEALTH PROFESSIONAL, by J.V. Stewart
PREPARING FOR MEDICAL PRACTICE MADE RIDICULOUSLY SIMPLE, by D.M. Lichtstein
MED'TOONS (260 humorous medical cartoons by the author) by S. Goldberg
CLINICAL RADIOLOGY MADE RIDICULOUSLY SIMPLE, by H. Ouellette and P. Tetreault
NCLEX-RN MADE RIDICULOUSLY SIMPLE, by A. Carl
THE PRACTITIONER'S POCKET PAL: ULTRA RAPID MEDICAL REFERENCE, by J. Hancock
ORGANIC CHEMISTRY MADE RIDICULOUSLY SIMPLE, by G.A. Davis
CLINICAL CARDIOLOGY MADE RIDICULOUSLY SIMPLE, by M.A. Chizner
PSYCHIATRY ROUNDS: PRACTICAL SOLUTIONS TO CLINICAL CHALLENGES, by N.A. Vaidya and M.A. Taylor.
PATHOLOGY MADE RIDICULOUSLY SIMPLE, by A. Zaher
CLINICAL PATHOPHYSIOLOGY MADE RIDICULOUSLY SIMPLE, by A. Berkowitz
ORTHOPEDICS MADE RIDICULOUSLY SIMPLE, by P. Tétreault and H. Ouellette
ATLAS OF ORTHOPEDICS, by P. Tétreault, H. Ouellette, and S. Goldberg
ANATOMY OF THE SOUL, by S. Goldberg
IMMUNOLOGY MADE RIDICULOUSLY SIMPLE, by M. Mahmoudi
CLINICAL BIOSTATISTICS MADE RIDICULOUSLY SIMPLE, by A. Weaver and S. Goldberg

Try your bookstore. For further information, write MedMaster, P.O. Box 640028, Miami FL 33164, or see http://www.medmaster.net. Email: mmbks@aol.com.